为你解答：
居家生活健康手册
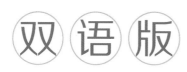

主　审　曾繁典　杜　光　宋启斌
主　编　邹　海
副主编　郭亚楠　朱　彪　牟晓洲
编　者　（以姓氏笔画为序）

王　勇　宁波市第一医院

毛美娇　上海中医药大学附属龙华医院

从恩朝　上海市精神卫生中心

朱　彪　复旦大学附属肿瘤医院

牟晓洲　浙江省人民医院

李方方　复旦大学附属肿瘤医院

李新艳　上海市公共卫生临床中心

余丽华　浙江大学医学院附属第一医院

邹　海　复旦大学附属肿瘤医院

宋宏伟　上海市中医医院

张　俊　上海中医药大学附属龙华医院

张忠伟　复旦大学附属肿瘤医院

张带荣　《医药导报》编辑部

陈颖颖　厦门大学附属中山医院

陈臻瑶　复旦大学附属肿瘤医院

郑毅隽　复旦大学附属肿瘤医院

郭亚楠　上海交通大学医学院附属仁济医院

郭勤浩　复旦大学附属肿瘤医院

彭小平　南昌大学第一附属医院

秘　书　张　俊　陈臻瑶

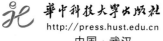
华中科技大学出版社
http://press.hust.edu.cn
中国·武汉

内 容 简 介

　　本书是由专业医生构成的"为你解答"科普团队，以一问一答的方式编写而成。全书共分为两大部分，第一部分为居家生活中常见问题的解答，如胃该怎么"养"、发现淋巴结肿大怎么办、心肺功能锻炼、心理问题如何疏导、高血压相关知识等，以深入浅出的语言为广大群众普及专业的医学健康知识。第二部分为医学人文故事介绍，记录真实的临床暖心小故事，让大众理解医生面对患者时的情景，以及具体的临床诊疗过程。

　　本书力主轻松活泼，附有大量精美的原创图片和视频，可以作为大众科普图书，供广大读者阅读。

图书在版编目 (CIP) 数据

　　为你解答：居家生活健康手册：双语版：汉英对照 / 邹海主编 . —武汉：华中科技大学出版社，2022.12

　　ISBN 978-7-5680-8958-6

　　Ⅰ . ①为… 　Ⅱ . ①邹… 　Ⅲ . ①健康教育－手册－汉、英 　Ⅳ . ① R193-62

中国版本图书馆 CIP 数据核字 (2022) 第 234993 号

为你解答：居家生活健康手册（双语版） 　　　　　　　　　　　　　邹　海　主编
Wei Ni Jieda: Jujia Shenghuo Jiankang Shouce (Shuangyu Ban)

策划编辑：蔡秀芳
责任编辑：曾奇峰
封面设计：廖亚萍
责任校对：刘小雨
责任监印：周治超

出版发行：华中科技大学出版社（中国·武汉）　　　电话：(027)81321913
　　　　　武汉市东湖新技术开发区华工科技园　　　邮编：430223
录　　排：华中科技大学惠友文印中心
印　　刷：湖北恒泰印务有限公司
开　　本：787mm×1092mm　1/16
印　　张：11.75
字　　数：154 千字
版　　次：2022 年 12 月第 1 版第 1 次印刷
定　　价：52.80 元

主编介绍

邹海，《医药导报》杂志编委，iMeta 青年编委。2022 年借助《医药导报》《新民晚报》等新媒体平台，建立了以医学科普为主的"为你解答"科普团队，为了市民在居家期间健康生活，适时发布有关健康的相关知识。获得 2020 年上海市人才发展资金、2020 年上海市"医苑新星"青年医学人才培养资助计划资助。主攻方向：呼吸危重症规范化诊治，肿瘤相关危重症诊治，常见疾病的科学预防及治疗。

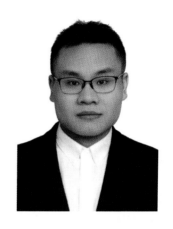

2018 年 11 月，获共青团浙江省委"最美 90 后"荣誉称号。作为主要参与者参与的项目"围手术期优质护理管理模式的建立和应用"获浙江省科学技术进步奖三等奖。2020 年 2 月，作为上海第四批援鄂医疗队队员，在一线火线入党，所在的 ICU 团队获"全国卫生健康系统新冠肺炎疫情防控工作先进集体"称号，本人获"复旦大学抗击新冠肺炎疫情先进个人"荣誉称号。2022 年 6 月，担任复旦大学附属肿瘤医院支援上海市公共卫生临床中心成员，获"抗击新冠肺炎疫情卓越个人及先进党员"荣誉称号。为了响应党员支援倡议和落实"双报到"要求，主动联系街道党支部开展健康科普服务。主持国家自然科学基金青年科学基金项目 1 项，浙江省科技厅社会发展项目 1 项。发表肿瘤、呼吸危重症、临床药物相关研究 SCI 论文 30 余篇，H 指数 16。参编译著 1 部。申请发明专利 1 项。

序 一

早在 2016 年，我国已制定并开始实施《"健康中国 2030"规划纲要》。这一宏伟规划，将党和国家高度重视提高人民健康水平的意志，发展为推进健康中国建设的具体行动。人民健康水平的普遍提高，已成为中华民族伟大复兴，实现民族昌盛和国家富强的重要标志。

我国的健康中国建设，是一项涉及各行各业的浩大工程，其中大力提高民众科学文化素质和健康素质，是实施这一工程的重要措施之一。鉴于此，中华医学会于 2022 年 7 月开启"科普中国医疗健康"项目，号召和组织广大医务工作者在努力完成本职医疗预防专业工作的基础上，积极参与医药卫生科普工作，使医学科普成为强化国民健康理念、提升全民健康素养、实现"健康中国"伟大目标的有效途径。医务工作者应关切广大民众对健康知识的迫切需求，有针对性地开展医学科普，助力公众对当下社会存在的纷繁杂乱"健康信息"进行识别，使公众对不同信息有能力"去伪存真"，做到科学养生、合理保健、及时就医防病，实现对幸福生活的美好追求。

复旦大学附属肿瘤医院、《医药导报》杂志编委邹海医生，武汉大学人民医院肿瘤中心宋启斌教授，上海中医药大学附属龙华医院张俊医生，上海市中医医院宋宏伟医生等多位志同道合的临床一线工作者组成"为你解答"科普团队，他们在临床实践中发现和收集民众存在的医学困惑，以问答方式逐一解惑，这种"一问一答"的解惑问答在《医药导报》微信公众号和《新民晚报》发表后，深受大众欢迎，成为大众获取医学科普知识的新途经。这些有用的医学科普问答经"为你解答"科普团队的认真修定，汇集成册，以飨读者。

我国青年医务工作者积极参与健康中国建设，积极投入医学科普工作实践，我国医学科普队伍由此得以壮大。青年医务工作者这种以实际行动服务社会、服务人民、服务医学科普的行为，具有重大意义，可喜可贺！预祝青年医学科普团队更加深入民众、更多了解民情，工作精益求精，在医学科普领域，百尺竿头，更上一层楼。

华中科技大学同济医学院

序 二

没有全民健康，就没有全面小康，《"健康中国2030"规划纲要》中着重强调：普及健康生活，加强健康教育，塑造健康行为，提高全民身体素质。提高公众的医学科学素养是摆在我们医务工作者面前的一项迫切任务，是有效的疾病预防策略。医学科普是一项高层次、高难度、多学科、多手段、多创新的将医学知识再加工的过程，就是将医学科学知识、防病治病方法、医学保健措施和健康理念，通过多种手段和途径传播给公众，提高全民健康意识、提升健康素养、倡导健康生活，帮助公众在生活起居中更好地防病，指导需要就医的患者正确就医。

随着互联网的普及与发展，出现越来越多的单点及碎片化的健康知识，对于缺少临床专业知识的公众来说，普遍存在对这些知识的真伪判断难、理解难、运用难的问题。如何贴近公众，选择他们最关心的健康话题，解答他们在健康养生、防病治病中的疑虑，宣传倡导正确的健康理念，深入浅出地介绍医学最新进展等，是医学科普的选题方向和工作重点。本书编者结合各自专业领域，将临床知识转化为通俗易懂的文字以及形象的图片，图文并茂地展现在读者面前。本书生活化、大众化、社交化、场景化，内容严谨，语言通俗，可读性强，覆盖人群广，使读者可身临其境地与医务工作者对话，聆听治病就医的暖心小故事，在潜移默化中学习到医学健康知识，解决健康困惑，了解临床医务工作者的工作，倾听到他们的心声。

在大众对健康日益关注的新时代，医学知识也不再囿于特定的传播渠道，而是存在于每一个与健康资讯需求相关的生活场景中。本书的愿景是读者能通过医学科普，熟悉常见的医学知识，这对个人、家庭和社会均有裨益。推动医学科普，提升健康理念，守护健康生活，建设健康中国是我们的责任，也是我们追求的目标。

杜光

华中科技大学同济医学院附属同济医院
国家重大公共卫生事件医学中心

序 三

党的十八大以来，以习近平同志为核心的党中央把维护人民健康摆在更加突出的位置，全国卫生与健康大会确立了新时代卫生与健康工作方针。习近平总书记强调的"没有全民健康，就没有全面小康"，意义深远。健康是促进人的全面发展的必然要求，是经济社会发展的基础条件，是民族昌盛和国家富强的重要标志，构建全民的卫生健康服务体系，是筑牢共同富裕的根基，是利国利民、福惠苍生的百年大计。

普及健康科学知识，提高健康教育服务能力，是提高全民健康意识工作的重中之重，也是医务工作者义不容辞的使命。医学的任务早已不仅仅是看好病，还要预防疾病，提高社会的健康水平。在生产力高度发展、物质水平日益丰富的今天，医学更是一种健康文化。

在这一背景下，《为你解答：居家生活健康手册（双语版）》经过各位编者反复讨论选题，凝炼内容，立足于广大百姓最基础、最迫切的健康需要，响应践行党中央坚持把科学普及放在与科技创新同等重要位置的要求，旨在提升全民科学素质，最终编撰出版。

本书将专业的医学知识以通俗易懂的语言、生动的图画，呈现给大众，帮助读者获取有益的医学健康知识，守护自己和家人的健康，也极大地提高了医疗资源的利用率。本书的编者大多是我国高校附属医院出类拔萃的一线临床医生，书中每一篇作品都是他们在夜以继日的临床工作、医学前沿研究中积累的经验所凝炼的知识精华。

　　本书从选题策划、章节编制，到内容撰写，始终贯彻专业至上、即看即懂、即会即用的原则，其最大的特点就是从老百姓的角度，把他们在日常生活中最想问的问题，经常碰到但答案又不统一的问题，乃至茶余饭后养生保健的问题，尽可能地汇聚起来，让专家来到他们身边。读者与作者，是患者与医生，但更是贴心朋友。开卷有益，读者在轻松愉快地阅读时，医学健康知识也涓涓细流入心中。

　　医学科普是一项崇高而长远的社会事业，是现代社会文明发展的重要组成部分，更是新时代中国特色社会主义构筑全民健康总目标的基石与强有力工具，中共中央办公厅、国务院办公厅印发的《关于新时代进一步加强科学技术普及工作的意见》中提到："科学技术普及是国家和社会普及科学技术知识、弘扬科学精神、传播科学思想、倡导科学方法的活动，是实现创新发展的重要基础性工作。"希望通过本书的出版发行，读者能亲近地感受到医学专业，正确理解、接受医学知识，充实自己，惠及亲友，造福社会；读者能体会医者笔下流淌着的良苦用心。医疗的本质从来都是帮助而不是交易，是医者对患者的关怀和爱护，满怀仁心布施仁术，是我们每一位医者矢志不渝的追求。

武汉大学附属人民医院

前 言

《"健康中国2030"规划纲要》提出了健康中国建设的目标和任务。《国务院关于实施健康中国行动的意见》将"实施健康知识普及行动"列入15个专项行动的首要行动。行动目标是提高全民的健康素养水平。健康科普类图书是普及健康知识的有效途径之一,医务工作者是健康科普的主力军,承担着大力开展医学健康知识普及、推广文明健康生活方式、引导人民群众提高自我防护和健康管理能力的重要任务。

公众渴求健康保健知识,但往往被虚假科普误导,他们希望身体健康,但又经常出现两种极端现象:有人身体不舒服,自己做医生,或迷信保健品广告;有人过于珍惜自己的生命,三天两头跑医院。如此等等反映出我们离科学的健康素养还差很远。传播正确的健康知识,引导大众进行合理的健康管理以及慢性病预防,十分必要,非常重要。在日常居家生活中,遇到健康问题该如何早识别、早预防、早干预,是公众关注的焦点,提高对健康的认识力、对健康宣传的判断力、培养健康知识的阅读理解力是提高公众健康素养的关键,也是进行健康科普的核心要素和任务。

基于此,我们组建了由专业医生构成的"为你解答"科普团队,以一问一答的方式,聚焦公众关注的健康热点、常见病、高发病、慢性病等,同时重在扫除健康盲区,纠正健康误区。书中插入大量精美的原创图片和视频,以提高公众的阅读体验,以此传播健康知识,传递养生智慧。

本书共分为两大部分。

第一部分为居家生活中常见问题的解答，如心肺功能锻炼、发现淋巴结肿大怎么办、心理问题如何疏导、中医养生以及常见慢性病的管理，以深入浅出的语言为广大群众普及专业的医学健康知识。

第二部分为医学人文故事介绍。通过一线临床医生的视角，记录真实的临床故事，让大众理解医生面对患者时的情景，以及具体的临床诊疗过程，以建立和谐的医患关系。

本书的撰写受到上海市人才发展资金，上海市"医苑新星"青年医学人才培养资助计划的资助。衷心感谢团队成员倾尽全力保证本书的严谨性和实用性。衷心感谢华中科技大学同济医学院曾繁典教授、华中科技大学同济医学院附属同济医院杜光教授、武汉大学附属人民医院宋启斌教授为本书审稿并作序！衷心祝愿读者开卷有益，能从一个新的视角去认识和理解个人和家庭的健康问题以及医患关系。让我们携手共同维护生命健康，为实现健康中国建设的目标和任务而努力！

在浩瀚无垠的健康知识海洋中，本书内容上难免有不足之处，还望广大读者谅解！由于医学科学的突飞猛进、网络技术的日新月异，本书的推荐意见以及内容不可避免地会有时效性。我们将随着时代科学技术的进步和发展，不失时机地修正、补充和完善本书的内容。

邹　海

目　录

第一部分

第二部分

Table of Contents

Part I

Part Ⅱ

第一部分

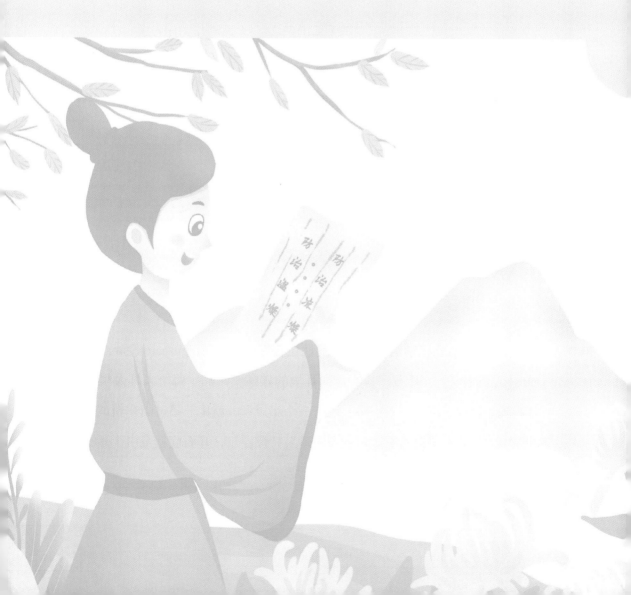

1、耳石症，一种常见的耳源性眩晕疾病

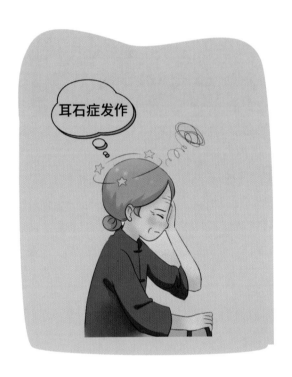

科普视频：
什么是耳石症

Q： 什么是耳石症？

A： 耳石症，学名叫良性阵发性位置性眩晕（benign paroxysmal positional vertigo，BPPV）。耳石，其实是内耳里的碳酸钙结晶。每个人耳朵里都有一层耳石膜，就像一层鹅卵石小路，还有三个半规管，就像三条过山车轨道。由于各种原因，鹅卵石般的耳石微粒会"脱落""漂浮"，耳石症就是由于耳石微粒从

掌管平衡的前庭器里"逃跑"，在半规管里滚来滚去"乘风破浪"造成的，患者处于特定的体位会诱发眩晕，天旋地转犹如"乾坤大挪移"。

Q: 有天旋地转的眩晕感，如何确定是不是耳石症呢？

科普视频：耳石症手法检查

A: 耳石症通过手法检查能够诊断，也能通过手法复位进一步确诊。典型表现是躺在床上时转头会有眩晕感。如果您有发作性的一过性眩晕，通常不超过1分钟，并且眩晕发作与体位变化有关，就需要考虑耳石症了。这种情况需至耳鼻咽喉科就诊。

Q: 居家生活期间得耳石症了怎么办？

科普视频：耳石症手法复位

A: 耳石症主要依靠手法检查确诊、手法复位治疗。

耳石复位治疗，即通过一系列沿特定空间平面的序贯式头位变动，使位于半规管管腔内或嵴帽表面的异位耳石颗粒按特定方向运动，经半规管开口回到椭圆囊而达到治疗目的。通俗来说就是通过改变头部特定的轨迹运动，引导"落跑"的耳石颗粒"回归正途"。

耳石症多可通过1～2次复位成功，部分患者需要经过多次手法复位。检查及手法复位过程中会诱发眩晕，小部分患者会有一过性恶心、呕吐、心慌等不良反应，可自行缓解。手法复位后适当的药物治疗或前庭康复锻炼可以加速前庭代偿。

Q: 手法复位后，还会复发耳石症吗？日常居家生活应如何避免复发？

A: 复位成功后短期内很少复发，小部分患者反复发作时，需与其他疾病鉴别，必要时行头颅磁共振检查排除中枢神经系统疾病。

研究表明，耳石症好发于 40～60 岁中老年人，女性发病率显著高于男性，耳石症的发作与骨质疏松、高脂血症、偏头痛等有一定相关性。日常生活中应戒烟，忌咖啡、酒、浓茶，限制盐分摄入，避免疲劳，避免强声强光刺激等。

Q： 头晕的时候"天旋地转"，肯定是耳石症吗？

A： 耳石症的特点是发作性的、体位相关性的眩晕感，但并非所有的眩晕都是耳石症。很多耳源性眩晕，如梅尼埃病、前庭型偏头痛、前庭神经炎等，都会引起"天旋地转"或者"摇摆感"。

Q： 眩晕的患者，可以首先去耳鼻咽喉科就诊吗？

A： 眩晕是一种表现，中枢性眩晕、颈性眩晕同样会引起这类症状。临床上我们最怕的是脑血管疾病、中枢神经系统疾病引起的眩晕，这种需要紧急处理。所以，眩晕的患者，还是建议首先至神经内科就诊。

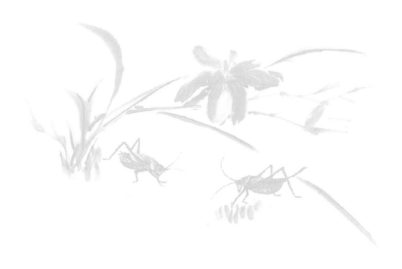

1.Otolithiasis, a common otogenic vertigo

Q: What is otolithiasis?

A: Otolithiasis is medically known as benign paroxysmal positional vertigo (BPPV). Otoliths, in fact, are calcium carbonate crystals in the inner ear. There is a layer of otolithic membrane in the ear, like a cobblestone path, and three semicircular canals, like roller coaster tracks. For various reasons, cobblestone–like otolith particles can "fall out" and "float". Otolithiasis is caused by otolith particles escaping from the vestibular apparatus, which is responsible for balance, and roll around in the semicircular canal. Specific positions will induce vertigo for the patients, and they will feel a spinning sensation as the world turns sideways.

Q: How can I determine whether or not I have otolithiasis if I feel a spinning sensation and have vertigo?

A: Otolithiasis can be diagnosed by manual examination and confirmed by canalith repositioning.Typical symptom includes dizziness when turning the head while lying in bed. If you have episodes of transient vertigo, usually less than 1 minute, and these episodes are associated with a change of position, you may have otolithiasis. It's advisable to visit the otolaryngology department.

Q: What should I do if I have otolithiasis when staying at home?

A: Otolithiasis can be diagnosed by manual examination and confirmed by canalith repositioning.

Canalith repositioning treatment is achieved by a series of sequential cephalometric changes along a specific spatial plane, making ectopic otolith particles located in the lumen of the semicircular canal or on the surface of the cupula move in a specific direction and return to the utricle through the opening of the semicircular canal. In simpler non-medical terms, this treatment guides the otolith particles that "ran away" "back on track" by moving the head in a specific trajectory.

Most patients with otolithiasis can be successfully treated by 1-2 treatments repositioning, but some patients need to go through multiple repositions. The examination and canalith repositioning may induce vertigo, and a small percentage of patients may have adverse reactions such as transient nausea, vomiting, and palpitation, which should remit spontaneously. Appropriate medication or vestibular rehabilitation exercises after canalith repositioning can accelerate vestibular compensation.

Q: *Can otolithiasis recur after canalith repositioning, and how should I avoid recurrence while staying at home?*

A: Recurrence is rare in the short term after successful repositioning. For a small percentage of patients, recurrent episodes need to be differentiated from other diseases. If necessary, a brain MRI should be performed to exclude the possibility of central nervous system diseases.

Research has shown that otolithiasis is more common in middle-aged and elderly people aged 40-60, with a significantly higher incidence in women than that in men, and that otolithiasis is associated with osteoporosis, hyperlipidemia, and migraines. In everyday life, it's advisable to stop smoking, avoid coffee, alcohol and strong tea, limit salt intake,and avoid fatigue, loud sound and light stimulation.

Q: If I feel a spinning sensation during vertigo, does that indicate I certainly have otolithiasis?

A: Otolithiasis is characterized by episodic and postural-related vertigo, but not all vertigo indicates otolithiasis. Much otogenic vertigo, such as Meniere's disease, vestibular migraine, and vestibular neuritis, can cause a "spinning" or "swaying" sensation.

Q: Can a patient with vertigo first go to an otolaryngologist?

A: Vertigo is a manifestation, and similar symptoms can also be caused by central vertigo and cervical vertigo. Clinically, we are most worried about vertigo caused by cerebrovascular diseases and central nervous system diseases; these require urgent treatment. Therefore, patients with vertigo are still recommended to visit the neurology department first.

2. 鼻出血的常见病因及居家紧急处理

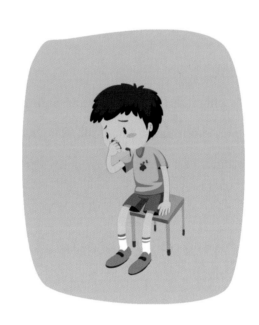

A: 鼻出血的常见原因包括局部因素和全身因素。

局部因素包括撞击、挖鼻或者用力擤鼻涕引起的鼻腔黏膜破损、鼻腔血管破损，或者鼻炎、鼻窦炎导致的黏膜糜烂，以及鼻中隔偏曲等解剖异常；鼻腔鼻窦的良、恶性肿瘤也可能导致鼻出血。

全身因素：最常见的就是我们在电视剧里经常看到的，因白血病等血液系统疾病导致的凝血功能障碍；高血压、冠心病的患者血管脆性增加，就像一根水管的管壁比较脆、水压又很高，一旦水管破损，就会有大量的血液溢出；发热、出血热、炎症、妊娠等导致毛细血管破裂，也容易引起鼻出血。

科普视频：
鼻出血的居家
处理

Q： 鼻出血时，如何紧急处理呢？

A： 一旦鼻出血，第一反应是不要慌，要保持冷静，情绪越紧张，血压越高，越会加重出血。

我们应该赶快坐下、身体前倾，用拇指和食指捏住两侧鼻翼（即鼻子前端软软的有弹性的部分）。捏鼻 5～10 分钟来压迫止血，在此期间，如果有血流到喉咙里，可以轻轻吐出鲜血，尽量避免误咽或误呛。

同时，我们可以去冰箱拿一些冰袋或者冷冻食品，敷在脖子或者脸颊旁边，通过冰敷使血管收缩、止血。冰敷时要记得裹一层毛巾，避免冻伤。如果有高血压且在家测量的血压较高，可以口服降压药。如果经过这些操作，还是没办法止血，需要去医院就诊。

Q： 小朋友鼻出血了，家长要怎么办呢？

A： 小朋友的鼻腔黏膜非常脆弱，有时候不小心被撞击或者挖鼻都容易导致鼻出血。

家长看到小朋友鼻出血，千万不能让小朋友仰头。可以把小朋友抱坐在怀里，由家长捏住鼻子压迫止血，同时叮嘱小朋友不要把血块咽下，否则容易呛到气管或者引起胃部不适。

Q： 鼻出血后，居家生活有哪些要注意的地方？

A： 鼻出血多因为血管或黏膜破损引起，愈合期需要数天到 1 周。在此期间，应避免挖鼻、用力擤鼻涕和剧烈运动。

饮食上，不能吃"热性食物"如火锅、辛辣食物、羊肉、山参等。以温冷软食为宜，避免吃过烫食物或者过度咀嚼食物导致再次出血。

生活习惯上，不能用力排便。排便时用力屏气很可能导致血管再次破裂出血。

如果反复发生鼻出血、鼻涕带血丝，建议至医院就诊，进行凝血功能检查、鼻内镜检查或 CT 检查等。

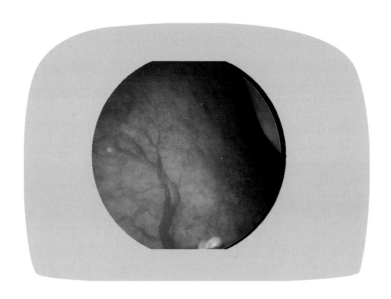

鼻腔毛细血管迂曲扩张引发鼻出血

2.Common causes of nosebleeds and emergency treatment at home

Q: What are the possible causes of nosebleeds when staying at home?

A: Common causes of nosebleeds include local and whole—body factors.

Local factors include damage of nasal mucosa or rupture of nasal blood vessels caused by injury, nose picking or forceful nose blowing, or mucosal erosion caused by rhinitis or sinusitis, or anatomical abnormalities such as nasal septum deviation. Benign and malignant tumors in the nasal cavity and sinuses may also cause nosebleeds.

In terms of whole—body factors, the most common is coagulation dysfunction due to leukemia and other blood system diseases, which we often see in TV series. Patients with hypertension or coronary heart disease have increased vascular fragility, just like when a water pipe with brittle walls experiences high water pressure. Once a blood vessel breaks, a large amount of blood will spill out. Broken capillaries due to fever, hemorrhagic fever, inflammation and pregnancy can also lead to nosebleeds.

Q: What is the emergency treatment for a nosebleed?

A: Once the nosebleed occurs, the first thing is not to panic and remain calm. The more nervous you are, the higher your blood pressure will be, which will aggravate the bleeding.

Sit down quickly, lean forward, and pinch the wing of the nose (the soft, elastic part at the front) with the thumb and index finger. Pinch the nose for 5–10 minutes to stop the bleeding with pressure. During this time, if there is blood flowing into the throat, you can gently spit out the blood. Be aware not to swallow or choke accidentally.

At the same time, you can go to the refrigerator to get some ice packs or frozen food, and put them on the neck or the cheek to constrict the blood vessels and stop the bleeding. Remember to wrap a towel to avoid frostbite when icing. If you have hypertension and your blood pressure is high when measured at home, you can take antihypertensive medication. If these measures do not stop the bleeding, it's advisable to go to the hospital.

Q: What should parents do when their children have nosebleeds?

A: Children's nasal mucosa is very fragile, so sometimes accidental bumps or nose–digging can easily lead to nosebleeds.

Parents should never let their children tilt their heads backward when their noses are bleeding. You can wrap the child in your arms and help pinch his or her nose to stop the bleeding while instructing him or her not to swallow the blood clot. Otherwise, it may lead to a trachea choke or cause discomfort in the stomach.

Q: *After a nosebleed, what should I pay attention to at home?*

A: Most nosebleeds are caused by broken blood vessels or mucosas and take a few days to a week to heal. During this time, you should avoid picking your nose, forceful nose blowing and strenuous exercises.

In terms of diet, you should not eat "heaty food" such as hot pot, spicy food, lamb and ginseng. It is advisable to eat soft foods that are balanced or cooling to avoid rebleeding due to excessive heat or excessive chewing.

In terms of daily habits, don't strain during bowel movements since straining may lead to re-rupture of blood vessels rebleeding.

If nosebleed or nasal discharge with blood occurs repeatedly, a hospital visit is advisable to conduct coagulation test, nasal endoscopy or CT scan.

3. 过敏性鼻炎，你需要知道的那些事

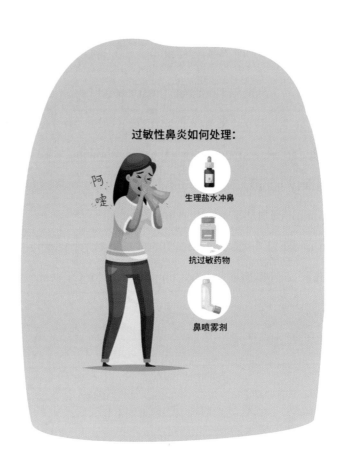

过敏性鼻炎如何处理：

生理盐水冲鼻

抗过敏药物

鼻喷雾剂

阿嚏

A: 这种现象很有可能是过敏性鼻炎。过敏性鼻炎的症状有鼻痒、打喷嚏、流清水样鼻涕，有时还有眼睛痒。过敏性鼻炎分为季节性和常年性。季节性过敏

性鼻炎一般发生在春季和秋冬季节，过敏原分别是花粉和蒿草等。常年性过敏性鼻炎全年都会有过敏症状，过敏原通常是尘螨。

Q： 过敏性鼻炎发作了，在家应该怎么处理呢？

A： 可以口服抗过敏药物，使用生理盐水冲洗鼻腔。如果有含抗过敏成分的鼻喷雾剂，也可以使用。

Q： 小孩子总是出现过敏性鼻炎，会与家里养狗有关吗？该怎么确定呢？

A： 宠物皮屑确实是常见的过敏原之一，如果想知道是什么原因引起过敏，可以进行过敏原检测。

过敏原检测包括过敏原皮试和血 IgE 检测。过敏原皮试比较快，但是需要近期没有服用过抗过敏药物。因使用抗过敏药物后，准确度会受到干扰。血 IgE 检测相对更为准确，但需要抽血检查。

Q： 我有过敏性鼻炎，居家生活需要注意哪些事项呢？

A： 过敏性鼻炎的患者，日常生活中，应注意避免粉尘多的环境，尽量保持生活环境洁净，定期除螨吸尘、勤晒被子。空调房间与外界温差不宜过大，否则容易加重打喷嚏、流鼻涕的症状。

如需外出，尽量戴口罩，避免因花粉或蒿草 / 种子诱发过敏性鼻炎。

过敏性鼻炎的患者，可以家中常备抗过敏药物和生理盐水。出行回家后建议用生理盐水洗鼻，可以清洁鼻腔、清除外界物质、缓解鼻腔症状。出现过敏性鼻炎的症状时，可以口服抗过敏药物或使用鼻喷雾剂。

3. Allergic rhinitis: what you need to know

Q: Is it because of allergic rhinitis if I sneeze and have nasal discharge when I clean or make the bed at home?

A: This is likely allergic rhinitis. Symptoms of allergic rhinitis include rhinocnesmus, sneeze, clear nasal discharge, and sometimes itchy eyes. Allergic rhinitis can be seasonal or perennial. Seasonal allergic rhinitis usually happens in spring and autumn/winter; allergens include pollen and artemisia. Perennial allergic rhinitis means that you will have allergy symptoms all year round; allergen is usually dust mite.

Q: What should I do at home when I have an allergic rhinitis episode?

A: You can take oral anti-allergy medication, use normal saline to rinse the nasal cavity, and use nasal sprays if available.

Q: My child always has allergic rhinitis. Can it be related to having a dog in the house, and how will I know this?

A: Pet dander is indeed one of the common allergens, and if you want to know what has caused the allergy, you can take an allergy test.

Allergy test includes allergy skin test and allergen-specific IgE test. An allergy skin test is faster but requires that no anti-allergy medication has been used recently, or else the accuracy may be affected. The allergen-specific IgE test is more accurate but requires a blood draw.

Q: I have allergic rhinitis. What do I need to be aware of when staying at home?

A: Patients with allergic rhinitis should try to avoid dusty environments, keep the living environment as clean as possible, and remove dust mites, vacuum and hang out the quilts regularly. The temperature difference inside and outside air-conditioned room should not be too large; otherwise, it can aggravate the symptoms of sneeze and nasal discharge.

If you go out, try to wear a mask to avoid allergic rhinitis induced by pollen or artemisia/seeds.

Patients with allergic rhinitis are recommended to always have anti-allergy medication and normal saline at home. After returning, wash your nose with normal saline, which can clean the nasal cavity, remove foreign substances and relieve nasal symptoms. When symptoms of allergic rhinitis onset, you can take anti-allergy medication or use nasal sprays.

4、鼾症，打呼噜也是一种病

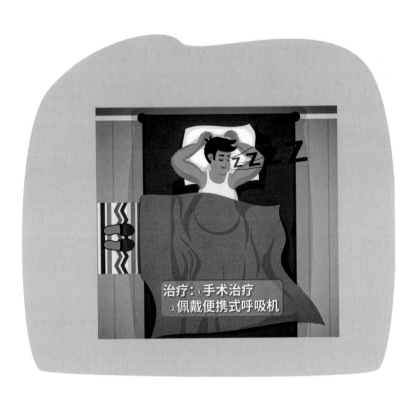

Q： 打呼噜也是一种病吗？

A： 打呼噜也可能是一种病，我们称之为鼾症。当打呼噜引起一定程度的呼吸暂停和缺氧时，就进阶为另一种疾病，称为阻塞性睡眠呼吸暂停低通气综合征。

Q: 阻塞性睡眠呼吸暂停低通气综合征，听起来很复杂，这种病严重吗？需要怎么判断呢？

A: 阻塞性睡眠呼吸暂停低通气综合征，是指夜间睡眠时，因为鼻腔或咽喉腔等上呼吸道狭窄，引发通气障碍或者呼吸暂停，导致血氧含量过低，因缺氧引发晨起乏力、白天嗜睡、记忆减退、顽固性高血压、性功能障碍等一系列伴随症状。

阻塞性睡眠呼吸暂停低通气综合征可以分为轻、中、重度，轻度者不要紧，但是这种病严重时可能会诱发严重的心脑血管损害，甚至引发猝死、呼吸心跳骤停。很多严重肥胖的人就是这样发生意外的。

肥胖、扁桃体肥大、下颌短小的人群容易发生这种疾病。当你的家人发现你打呼噜时有突然停下来，像是憋住了一样，过了几十秒又突然开始打呼噜的现象时，就很有可能是睡眠呼吸暂停，需要去医院做检查。

Q: 打呼噜需要做哪些检查呢？

A: 首先，需要评估体重指数（BMI），用体重（kg）/身高^2（m^2）计算而得，$18 \sim 24$ kg/m^2 为正常范围，小于 18 kg/m^2 是体重过轻，超过 24 kg/m^2 是超重，超过 28 kg/m^2 即为肥胖。其次，需要检查鼻腔和咽喉腔的通畅程度。最后，也是最重要的，需要进行多导睡眠监测（PSG）。多导睡眠监测是用仪器监测夜间的呼吸暂停、低通气、缺氧和打呼噜的程度，来判定是否达到了阻塞性睡眠呼吸暂停低通气综合征的标准，以及其严重程度。

Q: 打呼噜可以治疗吗？居家生活中有什么需要注意的吗？

A: 打呼噜是可以治疗的，可以通过手术治疗，或者佩戴便携式呼吸机治疗，具体选择哪种治疗方式需要完善检查后由医生进行评估。

居家生活中，需要戒除烟酒等容易加重鼻炎、咽喉炎的不良生活习惯。使用催眠镇静类药物容易引起咽喉肌肉松弛、加重阻塞症状，应尽量避免。建议减肥，减肥可以在一定程度上改善咽喉腔狭窄，还能减轻心肺负担。建议侧睡，侧睡可以减轻舌头后缀的情况，帮助呼吸道保持畅通。

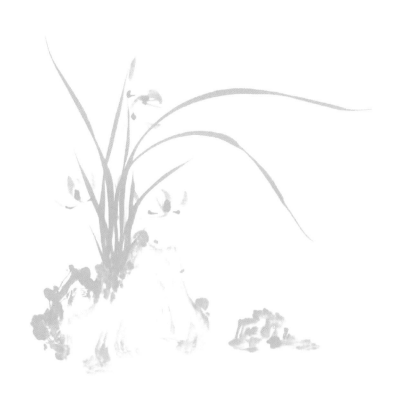

4.Snoring: it is an illness as well

Q: Can snoring also be a disease?

A: Snoring can also be a disease. When snoring causes some degree of apnea and hypoxia, it progresses to another condition called obstructive sleep apnea hypopnea syndrome (OSAHS).

Q: OSAHS sounds complicated; is this disease serious, and how can I tell?

A: OSAHS is a series of symptoms that occur at night when the upper airways, such as the nasal cavity or throat cavity, are narrowed, causing ventilation disorders or apnea, which leads to low oxygen levels in the blood. This can cause fatigue when waking up in the morning, drowsiness during the day, memory loss, resistant hypertension, sexual dysfunction, and other accompanying symptoms.

OSAHS can be divided into mild, moderate and severe cases. Mild ones are not serious, but severe ones may induce serious cardiovascular and cerebrovascular events, such as sudden death or sudden cardiac arrest. Many severely obese patients have had accidents like this.

People who are obese, have tonsillitis and have short jaws are prone to this disease. If your family finds you snoring and suddenly stopping, like holding it in, and then suddenly starting to snore again after about a minute, this is likely sleep apnea.

You need to come to the hospital for an examination.

Q: What examinations do I need for snoring?

A: First, a body mass index(BMI) evaluation is needed (i.e., weight/height squared in kg/m^2. The normal range is 18–24 kg/m^2; <18 kg/m^2 means underweight, >24 kg/m^2 means overweight, >28 kg/m^2 means obese). Next, the nasal and throat cavities need to be checked for patency. Finally, the most important is to take polysomnography (PSG), which is a procedure that uses machines to monitor the level of apnea, hypoventilation, hypoxia, and snoring at night to determine whether the criteria for OSAHS have been met and to determine what extent.

Q: Can snoring be treated, and is there anything I should be aware of when staying at home ?

A: Snoring can be treated either through surgery or by wearing a portable ventilator. A specific treatment plan needs to be evaluated by a doctor after a thorough examination.

In everyday life, be aware of quiting smoking and alcohol, and other bad habits that tend to aggravate rhinitis and pharyngitis. The use of sleeping and sedative drugs can cause relaxation of the throat muscles and aggravate the obstruction symptoms, which should be avoided. It is recommended that you try to lose some weight, which can improve the narrowing of the pharyngeal cavity to some extent and also reduce the burden on the heart and lungs. It is recommended that you sleep on your side, as it can reduce poor tongue positioning and help keep your airway open.

5、如何正确使用鼻喷雾剂及滴耳液

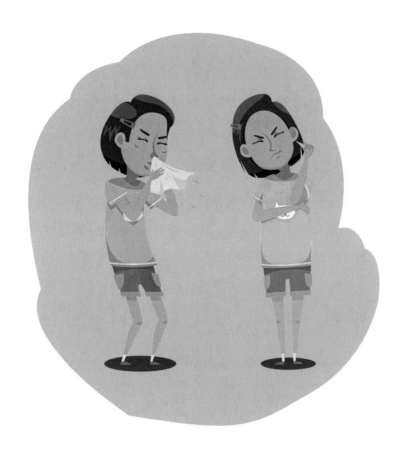

Q： 秋冬季节，我在家里经常觉得鼻子干怎么办？

A： 秋冬季节，天干物燥，很多人经常觉得鼻子干，甚至引起鼻出血，这个时候，我们可以使用家中常备的眼药膏或鱼肝油进行鼻腔护理。

可以把金霉素眼药膏、红霉素眼药膏挤在鼻腔前部，轻轻揉几下鼻子使药膏分布更为均匀。也可以将鱼肝油这种油剂类的胶囊戳破、滴在鼻腔里，进行润滑。如果有条件，可以购买护理型的生理盐水鼻喷雾剂，同样可以湿润鼻腔。

当然，如果使用1周以上症状没有改善，建议及时就医。

科普视频：
如何正确使用
鼻喷雾剂

Q： 我有鼻炎，日常生活中使用鼻喷雾剂有什么要注意的吗？

A： 鼻喷雾剂有很多种，如常见的鼻用糖皮质激素类药物、抗组胺类药物等。很多"网红鼻喷雾剂"含有血管收缩药物，虽然缓解鼻塞效果显著，但是不建议使用超过1周，否则容易引起药物性鼻炎。所以，大家使用鼻喷雾剂时，最好到医院去就诊开药，在医生的指导下合理用药。

使用鼻喷雾剂前，需要摘下瓶盖，如长期未使用，可对着空气喷1～2次，以获得均匀喷雾。喷鼻时，身体保持坐位、稍前倾，瓶身保持直立、稍向同侧眼角倾斜，喷一下即可，喷出的瞬间可配合吸气。

如使用鼻喷雾剂期间出现鼻干、鼻痛、鼻出血，可暂时停用药物并观察。

Q： 我晚上在家喜欢听歌，经常耳朵痒，忍不住挖，总有很多白色片状耳屎，这正常吗？

A： 经常戴耳机听歌导致耳痒，很有可能是外耳道湿疹。

外耳道湿疹是一种常见的耳部皮肤炎症，多由于过敏、反复挖耳刺激、长期佩戴入耳式耳机等引起。常见的症状是耳痒、耳流水、耳部皮肤脱屑，即你所说的"白色片状耳屎"很有可能是耳部皮肤脱落的皮屑。

在这种情况下，建议避免佩戴入耳式耳机，避免挖耳，避免摄入过敏性食物，如耳痒严重可以使用激素类湿疹药膏涂在耳道口，以止痒、促进恢复。

科普视频：
如何正确使用
滴耳液

Q： 我昨天去医院，医生说我有中耳炎，给我配了滴耳液，我忘记问怎么用了。

A： 我们常用的滴耳液是氧氟沙星滴耳液，建议每天早、中、晚三次，每次5～10滴。滴液前可以先把滴耳液在手心焐5分钟左右，因为过冷的滴耳液容易诱发眩晕。滴液的时候需要把脑袋歪过来，患耳朝上，滴耳液滴进去之后浸泡5～10分钟，我们称之为"耳浴"，然后把脑袋正过来，把流出的滴耳液自然擦去。滴耳液一般不建议连用超过1周。所以1周后务必停药、复诊。

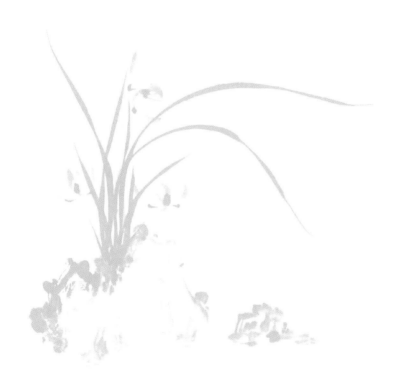

5.How to properly use nasal sprays and ear drops

Q: In the autumn and winter, my nose often feels dry when I am at home. What should I do?

A: In the autumn and winter, the weather can be dry. Many people often find their nose dry, and it may even lead to nosebleeds. You can use eye ointment or cod liver oil for nasal care.

You can squeeze gentamycin or erythromycin eye ointment on the tip of the nose and gently rub a few times to distribute the ointment more evenly. You can also break the capsule of the cod liver oil and drop it into the nasal cavity to moisten. If available, you can purchase a nursing normal saline nasal spray, which can also moisten the nasal cavity.

Of course, if the symptoms do not improve after more than 1 week of use, it is recommended to seek medical help.

Q: I have rhinitis. Is there anything I should be aware of when using nasal sprays in my daily life?

A: There are many kinds of nasal sprays, such as the common nasal glucocorticoids and antihistamines. Many "popular nasal sprays" contain vasoconstriction drugs. Although they are effective in reliving nasal congestion,it is not advisable to use them for more than 1 week; otherwise, they can cause drug–

induced rhinitis. Therefore, it is best to go to the hospital for prescribed medication and use it rationally with the guidance of a medical professional.

Before using the nasal spray, the cap needs to be removed. If it has not been used in a long time, spray it into the air 1–2 times to obtain an even consistency. Stay seated, and slightly lean forward. Hold the spray bottle upright, slightly tilted towards the eye corner on the same side of the nostril, and spray once. Inhale when you spray.

If nasal dryness, pain or bleeding occurs during the use of the nasal spray, temporarily stop the medication and observe.

Q: I like to listen to music at home at night, and my ears often itch, so I can't help but dig, and there is always a lot of white flaky earwax. Is this normal?

A: Ear itch after frequently listening to music using earbuds probably indicates ear eczema.

Ear eczema is a common inflammation of the ear skin, mostly caused by allergies, irritation due to repeated ear digging, and wearing earbuds for long periods of time. Common symptoms include ear itching, watering, and skin flaking, i.e., what you call "white flaky earwax" is most likely flaking skin.

In this case, it is advisable to avoid wearing earbuds, digging the ears,and eating foods causing allergies. If the itch is severe, use hormonal eczema cream on the ear canal opening to stop itching and aid recovery.

Q: I went to the hospital yesterday; the doctor said I had a middle ear infection and gave me the ear drops, but I forgot to ask how to use.

A: The ear drops we commonly use are ofloxacin ear drops. Use three times a day, in the morning, at noon and in the evening, with 5−10 drops each time. Before using, you can warm them in your hands for about 5 minutes, because ears drops that are too cold may induce vertigo. The drops should be applied with the head tilted over and the affected ear facing upwards; let the drops stay for 5−10 minutes, which is called an "ear bath". Then, turn your head back and wipe off the remaining drops from the ears. Ear drops are generally not recommended to be used for more than 1 week, so be sure to stop and get a follow−up.

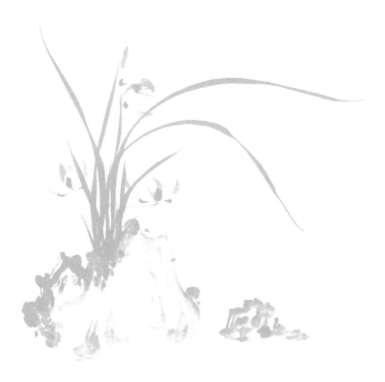

6、看古人秋季如何养生

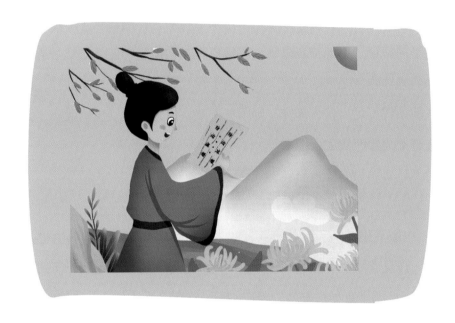

　　立秋是秋天的第一个节气，标志着炎热的夏天即将过去。立秋后，天高气爽、月明风清，气温由热逐渐下降。古代先贤总结了在立秋之后秋季的养生要点。

　　Q： 古人是如何在秋季生活起居的呢？

　　A： 《素问·四气调神大论》记录："秋三月，此谓容平。天气以急，地气以明，早卧早起，与鸡俱兴，使志安宁，以缓秋刑，收敛神气，使秋气平，无外其志，使肺气清，此秋气之应，养收之道也；逆之则伤肺，冬为飧泄，奉藏者少。"

Q: 古籍的这段记录我们如何理解呢？

A: 从字面意思看，秋季的三个月，谓之容平，自然界景象因万物成熟而平定收敛。此时，天气清肃，地气明静，人应早睡早起，和鸡鸣早起的活动时间相仿，天人合一，神志安宁，减缓秋季肃杀之气对人体的影响。形神俱守，以适应秋季容平的特征，不使神思外驰，以保持肺气的清肃功能，这就是适应秋令的特点而保养人体收敛之气的方法。若违逆了秋收之气，就会伤及肺脏，使提供给冬藏之气的条件不足。秋日未守，则阳气不藏，冬天就要发生飧泄病，大便泄泻清稀，并有不消化的食物残渣。

Q: 古籍的这段记录与我们现代生活有什么关联呢？

A: 中医养生是"天人相应"，即人与自然要和谐统一，养生也必须符合自然规律。在夏季因为日照时间较长，因此睡眠是"晚睡早起"，而到了秋季，阳气始降，作息规律要尽快改为"早睡早起"。立秋之后天气由热渐凉，进入了"阳消阴长"的过渡阶段，冷热变化快，人们易生病。早睡早起有利于提高人体免疫力，而早起适量的运动，可以使保持一天好心情的同时又能把每日的心肺功能储备积极地调动起来，良好的情绪可以有效减少疾病的发生。

Q: 除了"早睡早起"，我们还要注意什么呢？

A: 秋季往往是"燥"的，而我们的肺是"喜润恶燥"的，同时，暑性伤津耗气，夏季大量汗液的散发，也会导致体内津液相对亏耗，损伤肺津，因此入秋要特别注意养阴润肺燥。

这里的"燥"根据秋季温度的不同，又可分为"温燥"与"凉燥"，即"秋老虎"伴气候干燥是"温燥"，而秋尽冬来时则易发生"凉燥"。"温燥"与"凉燥"

的主要表现都有口、唇、鼻咽干燥，干咳无痰，皮肤干裂，大便秘结等；前者还有发热、出汗、口腔溃疡、鼻衄、口干渴等；后者则怕冷、头痛无汗、皮肤干痒、虽口唇干燥而不渴等。治疗上两者也是不同的。

根据"温燥"与"凉燥"的不同，我们平时养生时会选用不同的水果与蔬菜。

防治"温燥"可选梨、葡萄、猕猴桃、甘蔗、荸荠、番茄、萝卜、百合、鲜石斛。

防治"凉燥"可选柿子、石榴、广柑、苹果、白果、核桃、银耳、藕、胡萝卜、黑芝麻等。

因秋易"燥"，所以饮食还要少食辛味食物，如葱、姜、蒜、韭菜、辣椒等，在此基础上多吃些酸味、甘味食物，中医有"酸甘化阴"之说，可以润肺燥。

Q： 对秋季疾病的预防，我们要注意什么呢？

A： 第一，感冒、支气管炎。每到季节交替的时期有不少的人会被感冒缠身，而立秋之后天气也开始变得忽冷忽热，因此是感冒的多发季节，养生要多注意预防感冒。建议平时多注意根据天气的变化适当增减衣物，养成进门脱衣、出门增衣的习惯，早晚温差较大时尤然。

第二，胃病。要多注意胃病的预防，因为当人体遭受冷空气的袭击时会导致胃酸分泌过多，肠胃很容易出现痉挛，再加上立秋后食欲大增等因素，可导致胃病发作。建议除多注意保暖外，还要经常运动。饮食上也需要控制，做好少吃多餐、定时定量，避免过饱或过饥。

第三，过敏性疾病，如荨麻疹、哮喘、过敏性鼻炎。易过敏人群对环境变化敏感，环境适应能力差。一方面要加强体育锻炼，尤其是跑步、游泳、跳绳、骑自行车等有氧运动，以增强体质。另一方面尽量避免接触过敏原。尤其是体质较弱的老年人及儿童，应及时增减衣物，不可盲目坚持"春捂秋冻"之类的老话。

6.Regimen of ancient Chinese in autumn

The Beginning of Autumn is the first solar term in autumn, which signals the end of the hot summer. After the Beginning of Autumn, the weather becomes cool and crisp; the moon is bright, and the breeze is light; the temperature drops gradually. Ancient sages have summarized the key points of nurturing one's health in autumn.

Q: What is their daily routine like in autumn?

A: In the *Plain Questions—Great Theory on Spirit Regulation in the Four Seasons*, it was recorded: "The three months of autumn is the period of peace and maturation (rongping). The wind is strong, and the air over the earth is clear and bright. People go to bed early at night and get up early in the morning when they hear the crow of a rooster, to keep their spirit calm for separating themselves for the conquering sough of autumn, to astringent the spirit and energy internally to balance the autumn qi, and to ground the mind against anxiety to clear the lung qi. This is just the adaption to the autumn qi and the rules of nourishing the body. Disobeying the rule will impair the lung and bring about diarrhea after indigestion in winter due to insufficient qi storage."

Q: What does this record in the ancient text mean?

A: Literally, the three months of autumn are called rongping, meaning that the natural scenery calms down because it is the harvest season for all crops. At this time, the weather is clear and quiet. You should go to bed early and get up early, similar to the routine where roosters crow, so that you can be in unison with nature. The mind and spirit can be peaceful, thereby slowing down the impact of autumn chillness on your body. Protecting both the body and the spirit is the way to adapt to the characteristics of the three months of autumn, not letting the spirit or thoughts run away is the way to maintain the clearing of the lung qi. This is the method to adapting to the characteristics of autumn and maintaining the astringent qi in the body. If you disobey the autumn harvest qi, it will hurt the lungs, and making it not enough to provide the winter storage qi. If the autumn qi is not guarded, the yang qi has not been enough, then the winter will occur supper disease, diarrhea, clear and watery stool which contains food residues from indigestion.

Q: How does this record in the ancient text relate to modern-day life?

A: Traditional Chinese medicine (TCM) underscores "the adaption of the human body to the environment", that is, man should live in harmony with nature and health nurturing practices must also correspond with the patterns of nature. In summer, due to the long daylight hours, you can go to bed late and get up early; while in autumn, yang qi begins to decrease, and you should adjust your routine to going to bed early and getting up early as soon as possible. After the Beginning of Autumn, the weather gradually cools down, entering a transitional phase of "decreasing yang qi and increasing yin qi". With abrupt weather changes, it's easier to get sick. Going to bed early and waking up early is conducive to strengthening the immune system, and moderate physical exercise after getting up can not only boost your mood, but also mobilize cardiorespiratory reserves. Maintaining a good mood can effectively reduce illness.

Q: In addition to going to bed early and getting up early, what else should we pay attention to?

A: It's often "dryness" in autumn, and our lungs prefer to be moistened. At the same time, the summer heat hurts the body's fluids and consumes the qi, and a large amount of sweat will also lead to a relative deficiency of body fluids, thus damaging the lungs. So, we should pay special attention to nourishing the yin qi and moistening the lungs in autumn.

The "dryness" here can be divided into "warm dryness" and "cool dryness" based on the different temperatures in autumn, i.e., the weather during old wives' summer leads to warm dryness, while the weather at the end of autumn leads to cool dryness. The main manifestations of warm dryness and cool dryness are dry mouth, lip, nose and throat, dry cough without phlegm, dry and cracked skin, and constipation, while the former also manifests as fever, sweating, mouth ulcer, epistaxis, and thirst, and the latter also manifests as cold intolerance, headache without sweat, dry and itchy skin, and dry lips without thirst. The treatment of the two conditions is also different.

Based on the difference between warm dryness and cool dryness, we usually choose different fruits and vegetables in our regimen.

To prevent warm dryness,we choose pears, grapes, kiwis, sugar cane, water chestnuts, tomatoes, radishes, lily blubs, and fresh dendrobium.

To prevent cool dryness,we choose persimmons, pomegranates, mandarins, apples, ginkgo fruits, walnuts, snow fungus, lotus roots, carrots, and black sesame seeds.

As it's easy to experience dryness in autumn, choose less spicy and pungent foods such as onions, ginger, garlic, leeks and chili peppers. On this basis, eat more sour and sweet foods. In TCM, they can replenish the yin qi and moisten the lungs.

Q: *What should we pay attention to for the prevention of autumn diseases?*

A: Firstly, colds and bronchitis. During the change of seasons, many people often catch a cold, and after the Beginning of Autumn, the temperature starts to change abruptly, so it's more likely to catch a cold. So, in our regimen, we should pay more attention to preventing the cold. Pay attention to the weather changes and adjust the clothes we wear accordingly. Develop the habit of taking off and putting on layers when stepping inside and going outside, respectively, especially when the temperature varies a lot.

Secondly, gastric diseases. Pay more attention to preventing gastric diseases. Cold air lead to excessive secretion of gastric acid, making the stomach and intestines spasm; coupled with an increase in appetite after the Beginning of Autumn, and other factors, these can lead to the onset of gastric diseases. It is recommended to keep warm and exercise regularly. The diet also needs to be controlled: Eat less per meal and more meals on a set schedule and with portion control. Avoid overeating or starving.

Thirdly, allergic diseases such as measles, asthma and allergic rhinitis. People susceptible to allergies are sensitive to environmental changes and are less adaptable to the environment. On the one hand, increase physical activity, especially running, swimming, jumping rope, cycling and other aerobic exercises to enhance physical fitness. On the other hand, try to avoid contact with allergens. Especially the elderly and children, who are more susceptible should adjust what they wear in a timely manner. Do not blindly adhere to the old saying of "wearing more clothes in spring and less in autumn".

7.古语有云 "秋收冬藏" 之如何秋收冬藏

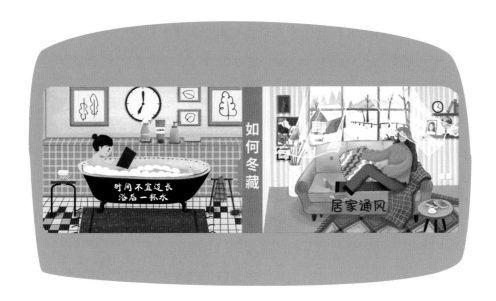

　　之前我们说到立秋，经过秋季之后，便是冬季。古语有云 "秋收冬藏"，出自西汉司马迁的《史记·太史公自序》："夫春生夏长，秋收冬藏，此天道之大经也。"其意思是秋季为农作物收获的季节，冬季则储藏秋天的成果以待来年需要，用于比喻一年的农事。那对应到我们人体，在冬季日常居家生活中如何封藏养生呢？接下来让我们一起看下。

Q: "冬藏" 与养生息息相关的来源。

A: 《素问·生气通天论》中记载："夫自古通天者，生之本，本于阴阳。天地之间，六合之内，其气九州、九窍、五脏、十二节，皆通乎天气。"其意思是自古以来，都以通于天气为生命的根本，而这个根本不外天之阴阳。天地之间，六合之内，大如九州之城，小如人的九窍、五脏、十二节，都与天气相通。中医学强调天人相应，人与自然和谐统一。同样，我们人体的调养也要顺应自然规律和四季交替法则，保养身体。"冬藏"的自然规律不仅是根源于天体的物理运行规律，更是传导引申出大自然植物与动物的生长规律，也就顺理成章地成为这个地球上人类重要的养生原则之一。

Q: "冬藏"的"藏"是什么？

A: 从中医学角度理解，冬季气候寒冷，寒气凝滞收引，真阳内守，气缓阳匿，易致人体气机、血运不畅，寒伤命门，体失濡养，而使许多旧病复发或加重。特别是那些严重威胁生命的疾病，如脑卒中、脑出血、心肌梗死等，发病率明显增高，所以冬季的养生要注意"储藏与温煦"。所谓"藏"最主要就是储藏和固护人体五脏的阳气。阳气主要有温煦、卫外、推动气血运行等重要作用，也是保持人体活力的精微物质。阳气在自然界主要指温热之气、升发之气，从子时开始生发，日中旺盛，日落衰减。在人体中，阳气晚上潜藏于体内，运行于五脏，因此晚上（特别是凌晨）是人体休养生息的时间。阳气通过各种气化活动完成人体与外界物质交换的主要过程，阳气活动上升于头面五官，扩散于躯干体表，使人精神焕发、意识清醒、感觉敏锐、温养形神，能随着外界环境变化做出相应调整，并驱使人体正常完成各种生物行为。

Q: 为什么要"冬藏"？

A: 在冬季，天地之气都闭藏起来了，人也应该闭藏起来。第一，是为了储备身体中的阳气，为第二年春天阳气生发做好准备，也就是为"冬藏"之后的"春生夏长"打下充足的物质与功能基础。第二，是为了保护身体中的阳气。冬天属于一年阳气此消彼长的下降期，是阴气最盈盛的季节。在日常生活中，户外天寒地冻，我们需要尽量减少外出活动，延长睡眠休息的时间，特别需要保证从子时至卯时的睡眠状态，以保护自身的阳气。《素问·四气调神大论》提到"冬伤于寒，春必病温"，也强调了冬季防寒和储藏阳气的重要性。人体如果出现阳气不足，则可能表现为畏寒肢冷、面色㿠白、神瘦倦怠、气短懒言、大便溏泄、小便清长、疼痛固化、活动不利等。

Q: 如何"冬藏"？

A: 第一，在冬季，宜早睡晚起，日出而作，顺应冬季的自然规律，保证充足的睡眠，有利于阳气潜藏、阴精蓄积。

第二，在穿着方面，应保证身体温暖不受寒，特别是在风大雪大的日子。衣着过少或过薄、肌肤皮毛暴露过多，或是环境温度过低，则易感冒而耗伤阳气；衣着过多或过厚、环境温度过高，则不利于阳气潜藏于内。

第三，在饮食方面，对于北方地区，冬季天气寒冷，宜食用牛肉、羊肉、生姜、当归之类的温补之品。对于长江以南地区，冬季气温较北方暖和，宜食用鸡肉、鱼类清补。对于高原山区，气候比较干燥，则宜食用甘润生津的果蔬、木耳、雪蛤、燕窝之类润补。相对平和的温性食物如南瓜、红枣、核桃、芝麻、小米粗粮之类均可食用。

第四，就是广为流传的服用膏方，冬令进补。依据中医辨证论治评估患者气血阴阳的状态进行调整，如对于慢性咳嗽、支气管哮喘、慢性阻塞性肺病、过敏性鼻炎，顽固性湿疹或是易感体质的患者，经过调整体质，可降低疾病急性发作的频率和程度。

Q: "冬藏"的时候需要注意什么？

A: 第一，在饮食方面，辛辣散表以及燥热温补之品不宜食用过多，前者容易辛散正气，后者可致壮火食气。同时，事物都有两面性，冬季能吃、能进补，但不能无节制，月盈则亏，水满则溢，否则就会导致肥胖症、冠心病等。因此，食补为本，但不宜过量。

第二，在服药方面，特别是服用膏方，必须由临床经验丰富的医生根据中医理法方药和君臣佐使的原则，在复方汤剂基础上，按人的不同体质、不同临床表现综合辨证而配制，一人一方，个体化配制。特别要注意的是，不同的人群体质不同，有寒热虚实之别。少年多阳气正盛，可以重调阴阳而轻补气血，以和为主。对于中年人群，则重固护脾胃生化之源，根据身体状态先建中土，后滋肾水。对于老年人群，则以养藏为主。冬季气温变化大，高血压、冠心病患者要注意保暖和规律用药，同时也可配合柔和锻炼方式，如太极拳、八段锦，旨在通过导引调动气血。

第三，在居家生活中，首先，如今冬季为保暖而常常窗户紧闭不通风，加上室内有空调、地暖装置等，容易造成环境温度过高，空气流通不佳，如果穿得过多过厚，常常会出现口干舌燥、面部潮红的表现，则提示阳气郁而化火，需要保持室内空气的流通以及适当饮水补充水分。其次，冬季天气寒冷，很多人喜欢蒙头睡觉，这会由于氧气不足而导致呼吸困难，不仅不能帮助人体保养热气，还会影响到身体健康。最后，冬季洗澡不宜太频繁。热水洗澡后，周身腠理疏通，毛窍开放，有发汗耗气的作用，也增加了寒气入里、侵袭六经的风险，因此洗澡时间也不宜过长、次数不宜太频繁，洗后慢慢地饮一杯温开水，以补充洗澡"丢掉"的水分。

7.How to "harvest in autumn and store in winter" as the old saying goes

We talked about the solar term "the Beginning of Autumn" earlier, and the winter comes after the autumn. The ancient saying "harvest in autumn and store in winter" is from *Shiji—Taishigong Zixu* by Sima Qian in the Western Han Dynasty: "Generate in spring, grow in summer, harvest in autumn and store in winter. This is the great scripture of heaven." It means that autumn is the harvesting season, and winter is the time to store the fruits of autumn for the next year. This is a metaphor for this year's farm work. What about our body? How do we seal and store to nourish our body? Let's take a look together.

Q: The source of "storing in winter" being closely related to the regimen.

A: In the *Plain Questions—Generative Qi Communicating with Nature*, it was recorded: "The communication with heavenly qi has been considered fundamental to life since ancient times, which is in turn based on yin and yang. Between the heaven and the earth, within the six directions of the universe, qi exists in nine states, nine orifices, five zang viscera and twelve joints of the body, all of which communicate with the heavenly qi." It means that since ancient times, the fundamental of life has been the communication with heavenly qi, and it is based on yin and yang. Between the heaven and the earth, within the six directions, everything as large as the nine states of the country, or as small as the nine orifices, five zang viscera, and twelve joints of humans communicates with heavenly qi. TCM emphasizes the correspondence and harmony between man and nature. Likewise, the human body should be maintained according to the laws of nature and alternating seasons. The natural law of "storing in winter" is not only rooted in the physical operation of the celestial bodies, but also extends to the growth pattern of the plants and animals in nature, which has logically become one of the important principles of human health on the earth.

Q: What does the "storing" of "storing in winter"?

A: From the perspective of TCM, due to the cold weather in winter, the coldness coagulates and stagnates; so, the real yang qi is guarding inside; when the yang qi slows down and is hidden, the flow of qi and blood is not unobstructed in the body, and the coldness hurts the vital gate, causing the body to lose nourishment, making many old diseases recur or worsen. Especially for those serious life-threatening diseases, such as stroke, cerebral hemorrhage and myocardial infarction, the incidences are significantly higher. So, when nourishing in winter, pay attention to "storing and warming". "Storing" refers to preserving and protecting the yang qi in the five zang viscera in the human body. Yang qi mainly plays an important role in warming, defending and promoting the movement of qi and blood. It is also the essence that keeps the body alive. Yang qi in nature mainly refers to the warm and hot qi, and the qi of ascension and development, which begins to generate at the hour of the sunrise, flourishes in the middle of the day and dwindles at sunset. In the human body, yang qi is latent in the body at night and runs through the five zang viscera; so, the night, especially the early morning, is the time for the body to recuperate. Yang qi completes the main process of material exchange between the human body and the outside world through vaporization. Yang qi rises in the five senses on the head and face and spreads on the surface of the torso so that people are refreshed, conscious, sensitive, warm and nurtured, and can make corresponding adjustments with changes in the external environment and drive their body to complete various biological behaviors normally.

Q: *Why "storing in winter" ?*

A: In winter, the qi in the heaven and earth are all closed and hidden. People should also conceal their spirit. Therefore, firstly, it is to reserve the yang qi in the body to prepare for the generation of yang qi next spring. It also accumulates sufficient material and functional basis for the generation in spring and growth in summer after the storage in winter. Secondly, it is to protect the yang qi in the body. Winter is the time of the year when yang qi declines, and yin qi is the most abundant. In our everyday life, when it is cold outside, we need to minimize outdoor activities and increase the time for rest and sleep, especially to ensure that we are asleep 23:00 — 7:00 the next morning to protect the yang qi in the body. The *Plain Questions — Great Theory on Spirit Regulation in the Four Seasons* mentioned that "if people are attacked by winter cold, they will lose their vigor in spring", which also emphasizes the importance of protecting against cold and storage of yang qi in winter. If the human body has yang deficiency, it may manifest as fear of cold, cold limbs, pale face, lethargy, shortness of breath and not wanting to talk, loose stools, clear and long urine, solidified pain and inability to exercise.

Q: *How to "storing in winter" ?*

A: Firstly, in winter, it is advisable to go to bed early, get up late, and start working at sunrise, in accordance with the patterns in nature. Ensuring sufficient sleep is conducive to the hiding of yang qi and the accumulation of yin essence in the body.

Secondly, in terms of clothes, ensure that the body is warm and not cold, especially on windy and snowy days. Dressing too lightly will cause too much exposure of the skin and hair, or if the room temperature is too low, it will be easier to catch a cold or deplete the yang qi. On the contrary, wearing too much and too thick, or staying in an environment with a temperature too high is not conducive to yang qi being hidden inside.

Thirdly, in terms of diet, for those in northern China, it's beneficial to consume warming tonics such as beef, mutton, ginger and angelica in the cold winter. In areas to the south of the Yangtze River, whose winter is warmer than that of the north, it's beneficial to consume moistening tonics such as chicken and fish. For the highland mountain areas that are relatively dry, it is appropriate to eat sweet and moist fruits and vegetables, fungus, hasma and bird's nest as moistening tonic. You can consume relatively neutral and warm foods such as pumpkin, dates, walnuts, sesame seeds, millet and other coarse grains.

Fourthly, it is common practice to take poultices as winter tonic. It will be adjusted based on the evaluation of the patient's qi, blood, yin and yang through symptom differentiation. Through constitution adjustment, the frequency and extent of acute onset can be reduced for patients with chronic cough, bronchial asthma, chronic obstructive pulmonary disease, allergic rhinitis, persistent eczema or susceptible constitution.

Q: *What to pay attention to when "storing in winter"?*

A: Firstly, in terms of diet, it is not advisable to consume too much spicy or hot food, as the former can easily disperse the qi, and the latter can lead to hyperactive fire consuming qi. At the same time, there are two sides to everything. Winter is a good time to eat and take tonic, but do not overdo it. The moon waxes only to wane, and water brims only to overflow. Otherwise, it can lead to obesity and coronary heart disease. Therefore, tonic food is essential but should not be over-consumed.

Secondly, in terms of taking medication, especially ointment, must be prepared by a clinically experienced physician according to the principles of TCM theory and prescriptions and the "monarch minister assistant guide" principle for compound tonics, considering the different constitution and clinical manifestations of each person to provide a prescription for each person. Special attention should be paid to the fact that different groups of people have different constitutions, which should be treated differently. Most teenagers have abundant yang qi, so they can focus on regulating yin and yang while lightly supplementing qi and blood, with harmony as the main focus. For the middle-aged population, the focus is on protecting the biochemical source of the spleen and stomach by first building up the middle foundation and then nourishing the kidney fluid based on their current physical state. For the elderly population, the main focus is on nourishing and storing. Patients with hypertension and coronary heart disease should keep warm and continue to take medication regularly in winter when there are large temperature fluctuations. It can also be combined with gentle exercise modalities, such as Tai Chi and Baduanjin, which are designed to mobilize qi and blood through Daoyin.

Thirdly, when staying at home, first of all, nowadays, winter heating often leads to closed windows without ventilation, coupled with indoor air conditioning and floor heating devices. It's easy to lead high indoor temperature and poor ventilation. If you wear too many layers, you will often feel dry and thirsty, with red cheeks. This is a signal that yang qi has been depressed and transformed into fire, and better circulation and more water intake are needed. Also, in the cold winter, many people like to cover their faces when they sleep. In fact, sleeping with your face covered will cause breathing difficulties due to insufficient oxygen, which not only does not help the body maintain heat, but also negatively affects health. Finally, avoid bathing too frequently in winter. After a hot water bath, the skin, the hair and the orifice are all open,not only leading to a sweating effect and a depletion of qi, but also increased the risk of cold into the six channels, so the bath should not be too long or too often. Slowly drink a glass of warm water afterwards to replenish "lost" water.

8、胃该怎么"养"

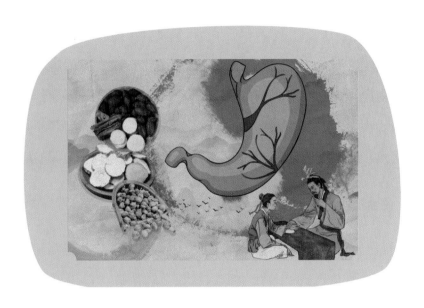

随着我国社会发展水平的不断提高、生活条件的日益改善，我们在日常的饮食和生活节奏上，已经比改革开放以前发生了翻天覆地的变化。在大都市里生活的人群，饮食谱越来越丰富，作息规律也千奇百怪，"乱象丛生"，形成了很多不良的饮食习惯，最终导致不同程度的胃部不适，甚至胃部疾病，直接影响了人们的生活质量。传统中医对于胃病，重养胜过重治，对于寻找胃病规律，重因胜过重症，那么对于我们的胃，到底应该怎么"养"呢？

Q: 胃的生理功能有哪些？

A: 胃主受纳水谷。受纳是接受和容纳的意思。胃主受纳是指胃接受和容纳水谷的作用。饮食经食管入胃腑，这一过程称为受纳。《灵枢·玉版》中提到："人之所受气者，谷也。谷之所注者，胃也。胃者，水谷气血之海也。"人体所有的生理活动以及气血津液的化生，都依赖摄入食物的营养，胃的受纳功能则是其腐熟功能的基础，如果胃的受纳功能下降，则会出现纳呆、胃脘胀闷、反胃等胃部不适的症状。

胃主腐熟水谷。腐熟是食物经过胃初步消化形成食糜的过程，《难经·三十一难》中提到"中焦者，在胃中脘，不上不下，主腐熟水谷"。被酸化挤磨的食糜下行于小肠，与后续的消化液混合进行营养摄取，形成了胃肠的消化吸收。如果胃的腐熟功能下降，就会出现胃脘疼痛、嗳腐食臭等食滞胃脘的症状。

Q：决定胃功能状态好坏的重要因素有哪些？

A： 胃作为我们人体消化食物的重要器官，它的工作状态受多种因素的影响，可综合归纳为以下三大因素：饮食、冷暖以及情绪。

在饮食方面，最为重要的是要有节制，在经济条件越来越好的今天，暴饮暴食已经成为各种餐桌上的普遍现象，过分的饱胀不仅会透支胃酸的分泌功能，也会严重抑制胃动力，从而诱发胃部的各种不适，也会损伤胃的正常生理功能，甚至生理结构。过分的饥饿也很伤害我们的胃，在日常生活中，人们往往会因为忙碌而错过饭点，有时甚至连续两顿，亦或是因为熬夜而直接睡过早餐的饭点，这时在正常生理周期下分泌的胃酸会因为没有食物中和其酸性而对固有胃壁、胃体产生腐蚀作用。如果长期过饥，还会反射性地影响正常的胃肠蠕动，减弱胃的腐熟功能。我们就餐时应该细嚼慢咽，让食物在口腔内的粗加工尽可能完整，从而减轻胃的受纳压力。

在冷暖方面，我们最需要注意的就是胃部的保暖，这里的保暖也分为两个层面，首先应注重人体外部环境的保暖，春秋季节冷暖交替的时候需要适当增减衣被，在夏季睡在空调房间的时候，腹部需要一定程度的遮盖，避免空调直吹，在家中时着袜穿鞋，避免寒从脚底而入。其次要尽量避免进食生冷的食物，包括冰牛奶、鸡蛋白、绿叶菜、水果、贝壳类的海鲜河鲜以及其他含水量高的食物。中医认为这些食物性寒，需要避免过多食用。

在情绪方面，应保持情志舒畅、乐观开朗，避免紧张焦虑以及急躁发怒或是抑郁的状态，这些负面的情绪状态，对胃的正常生理功能的影响相当明显。如果长期生活在这些不良的情绪之下，甚至会给胃带来不可逆转的实质性病变。

Q：胃食管反流该注意哪些？

A： 经常会有人说到，我怎么总是会有烧心、反酸、嗳气的症状，严重影响日常的饮食、起居以及社交。这类症状其实都属于胃食管反流的典型表现，同时还包括胸骨后疼痛、吞咽困难、咳嗽等临床表现。本病发病机制复杂、症状多样，迁延难愈，常常反复发作，甚者可发展成为反流性食管炎。从目前的临床及基础研究发现，不合理的饮食习惯、生活方式将直接决定本病的诱发和转归。

胃食管反流有以下五大需要重点注意的饮食禁忌，如果你有明显主症，必须要注意避免和纠正。

（1）避免饮酒，特别是高度酒和烈性酒。

（2）避免甜味道的食物，包括各种蛋糕、松软的面包（富含起酥油）、夹心饼干、各类蜜饯、甜味道的饮料、含糖量很高的水果（葡萄、哈密瓜、芒果、荔枝等）、糖分较大的红烧肉。

（3）避免油脂含量高的食物，比如油炸烧烤食品、肥肉、各类坚果（花生、瓜子、开心果、杏仁、夏威夷果、芝麻、核桃）。

（4）避免各类高热量的荤菜，如猪肉、牛羊肉、动物内脏等。

（5）避免刺激性较大的食物，如辛辣食物、浓咖啡、浓茶等。

另外还需要注意情绪的舒畅和平缓，避免过大的波动和紧张焦虑，保持乐观。避免在睡前2小时进食。已经诊断为胃食管反流的患者，睡觉时可适当抬高床头以缓解夜间症状，同时尽量避免弯腰或者前倾后仰这类剧烈改变上半身体位的动作。

Q： 胃不好的人，是否应该多"补补"？

A： 很多朋友经常会这样问："我的脾胃功能不大好，吃东西消化能力差，稍微多吃一点就难受，大鱼大肉吃得再多再好，也不长肉，我是不是要补一补啊？"

已故的上海著名"国医大师"张镜人老先生说过："胃病的病人要慎用补药。"其中所指的补药就是我们传统意义上的补气中药，如人参（党参、太子参）、黄芪。脾胃功能不良的人，其受纳水谷和腐熟水谷的功能都会下降，如果使用补气药物，不仅很难即刻实现提高消化功能的目标，反而会增加胃的工作量，使更多的"气"停滞在胃内，传导运化更加不畅，从而加重胀闷不舒的症状。胃肠功能紊乱后，补进去的"气"还会乱窜，引起胃痛，甚至影响胃口，导致不思饮食。所以胃不好的人，尤其是急性期的患者，切忌乱用参芪枣之流的补药。纵使是"标准"的虚证患者，也一定需要经中医辨证论治，因人而异地诊疗，才能安全使用补药。

Q： 简易有效的养胃食疗方有哪些？

A： 我们的胃确实在大部分时间都是在"工作"的，如何通过吃，来让胃边工作边调养呢，给大家推荐如下几个简单的食疗方。

（1）用粳米和糯米，采用1∶1的比例混合煮粥，酌情代替三餐的主食来食用。如果长期虚寒腹泻，可以加入适量铁棍山药和芡实（鸡头米）。中医认为粳米和糯米都有补益中气、健脾益胃的作用，山药和芡实有健脾补肾、固涩养胃的功效，而且糯米性温，也符合胃喜温恶寒的生理特性。如果做成糯米类点心，对大多数人来说，容易产生不易消化的风险，改变烹饪方法，用糯米煮粥，就可以祛弊就利，获得良效。

（2）取山药9g、六神曲9g、谷芽9g、麦芽9g、甘草3g，入水煎煮，煮开后15分钟关火，去除药渣，再加入大米煮粥。对于经常出现餐后饱胀的胃病患者来说，是非常有效简便的食疗小方。山药健脾养胃，谷芽和麦芽消食和胃，此三者对于胃气的固护堪称"铁三角"；六神曲甘温入胃经，对于脘腹胀满、消化不良有奇效；甘草补中益气，缓急止痛。诸药相合，长期服用可以养胃健脾，改善消化功能。

（3）以木蝴蝶6g、凤凰衣9g，与大米同煮食用。本方适用于空腹胃痛，进食后好转的人，亦适用于各类胃、十二指肠黏膜糜烂、溃疡的患者长期保健食用。木蝴蝶乃紫葳科植物木蝴蝶的干燥成熟种子，有疏肝和胃生肌之功，可以治疗肝胃气滞的胃痛。凤凰衣，通俗的说就是鸡蛋壳的内膜，性平味甘，入肺、脾、胃经，有收敛生肌之效。二药疏理肝气，调和胃气，宣畅肺气，以起到护膜医疡的作用。

8.How to take care of the stomach

With the continuous social development in China, living standards have improved drastically. Our diet and pace of life have changed dramatically compared to those before the reform and opening up. People living in metropolitan areas have an increasing variety in their diet. Their daily schedule is also weird and chaotic, which leads to unhealthy eating habits and various stomach issues or even diseases in the end. This directly impacts the quality of life. For gastric diseases, TCM emphasizes recuperation over treatment; in search of the patterns of these diseases, TCM emphasizes the cause over the symptoms. So, how should we recuperate the stomach?

Q: *What are the physiological functions of the stomach?*

A: The stomach is the main acceptor of water and grain, which means its main functions are to accept and accommodate the food and drinks consumed. Accepting is the process where the food and drinks enter the stomach through the esophagus. *Lingshu — Yuban* mentioned: "The qi in human body comes from grains, and grains are accepted by the stomach. The stomach is the sea of water, grain, qi and blood." All physiological activities of the human body and the production of qi, blood and fluid depend on the nutrients from the food intake. The stomach's receptive function is the basis of its putrefaction function; if the stomach's receptive function decreases, there will be symptoms of stomach discomfort such as dullness, bloating and nausea.

The stomach is responsible for ripening water and grain. Ripening is the process where food is initially digested by the stomach to form chyme, as mentioned in the *Nanjing — Thirty-one Difficulties*: "The middle burner (zhongjiao) is in the stomach and is responsible for ripening and digesting the water and grain." The acidified and squeezed surimi then travels down to the small intestine, where it mixes with subsequent digestive juices for nutrient uptake, forming gastrointestinal digestion and absorption. If the gastric decomposition function decreases, symptoms of food stagnation in the stomach, such as pain in the stomach and epigastric region, belching and smelly food will occur.

Q: What are the important factors that determine the level of stomach function?

A: The stomach is an important organ for digesting food in the human body, and its function is influenced by many factors, which can be summarized as diet, temperature and emotions.

In terms of diet, the most important is everything in moderation. As the economic conditions have drastically improved, it is common to binge eat or drink. In fact, overeating will not only overdraw the gastric secretion function, but also seriously affect proper gastric motility. This can induce a variety of stomach discomfort,and damage the normal physiological function and even the physiological structure of the stomach. Starvation is also very harmful to the stomach. In everyday life, skipping a meal due to the hectic schedule, sometimes even skipping two meals in a row, or not waking up for breakfast due to staying up late can cause the gastric acid secreted in normal physiological cycles to erode the stomach and stomach wall because there is no food. Long-term starvation can also reflexively affect proper gastric motility and weaken the decomposition function of the stomach. Also, it's important to chew the food thoroughly before swallowing so that the rough processing is as complete as possible in the mouth, which can alleviate some pressure on the stomach.

In terms of temperature, the most important is to keep the stomach warm. There are also two aspects to this. One is the external environment of the body. At the change of season between spring and autumn, when the temperature changes greatly, adjust clothes and bedding accordingly. When sleeping in air-conditioned rooms in summer, use a cover to avoid direct air conditioning. Wear socks and slippers at home to avoid cold seeping in from sole of the feet. The other one is to try to avoid eating raw and cold foods, including cold milk, egg whites, leafy greens, fruits, shellfish and other foods with high water content. In TCM, these foods are considered cooling in nature and should not be consumed excessively.

In terms of emotions, try to stay in a good model, be optimistic and cheerful, avoid tension and anxiety, as well as impatience, anger or depression. These negative emotions can significantly impact the normal physiological function of the stomach. In the long-term, they can even bring irreversible substantial lesions to the stomach.

Q: What should I be aware of if I have gastroesophageal reflux disease (GERD)?

A: People often ask why they experience heartburn, acid reflux and burping, which seriously affects everyday life and social interactions. These symptoms are all typical of GERD. Other symptoms also include retrosternal chest pain, difficulty swallowing, and coughing. The pathogenesis of this disease is complex, with a variety of symptoms, and it is difficult to cure, as it often recurs and can even develop into reflux esophagitis. From current clinical and fundamental research, it is found that unhealthy eating habits and lifestyle will directly determine the predisposition and regression of this disease.

There are five major dietary restrictions for GERD that you need to pay close attention to. If you have clear primary symptoms, these should be followed.

(1) Avoid drinking alcohol, especially strong ones.

(2) Avoid sweet food, including all kinds of cakes, fluffy bread (rich in shortening), sandwich cookies, preserved fruits, sugary drinks, fruits that are high in sugar (grapes, cantaloupes, mangoes, and lychees), and braised pork cooked with a lot of sugar.

(3) Avoid foods with high-fat content, such as fried food and barbecue, fatty meat, and nuts (peanuts, melon seeds, pistachios, almonds, macadamia nuts, sesame seeds, and walnuts).

(4) Avoid meat dishes high in calories, such as pork, beef, lamb and organ meat.

(5) Avoid stimulating food, such as spicy food, strong coffee and strong tea.

It is also necessary to try to stay calm and comfortable, avoid excessive mood swings, tension and anxiety, and remain optimistic. Avoid eating 2 hours before bedtime. For those diagnosed with GERD, sleep with an elevated pillow to relieve nighttime symptoms; avoid drastic position changes in the upper body, such as leaning forward and bending backward.

Q: *Should people with stomach issues consume more tonics?*

A: Those people with low spleen and stomach function often ask whether they need to consume more tonics, since they have a weaker digestion, feel bloated easily after eating, and do not absorb much nutrient from even feasts.

The late Mr. Zhang Jingren, renowned "Master of TCM" in Shanghai, said that patients with stomach issues should be careful with tonics. The tonic herbs referred to therein are the traditional Chinese herbs that are used to nourish qi, such as ginseng (tangshen and heterophylly falsetarwort root) and milkvetch root. People with poor spleen and stomach function will have a reduced ability to accept and digest food. So, if you use medication that nourishes qi, not only will it be difficult to achieve the goal of improving digestive function, but also it will increase the burden on the stomach, causing more qi to stagnate, making the conduction and transportation of food more difficult, thus aggravating distention and discomfort. After gastrointestinal dysfunction, the qi that was introduced by the medication can also run amok, causing stomach pain and even affecting the appetite. Therefore, people with stomach issues, especially those in the acute stage, should not consume tonics such as ginseng, astragalus and dates. Even standard deficiency patients must be treated by herbalists based on syndrome differentiation on a case-by-case basis in order to consume tonics safely.

Q: *What are some easy and effective stomach remedies?*

A: Our stomach, indeed, is working most of the tie. How can we let it recuperate while working? The following remedies are recommended.

(1) Combine equal parts of japonica rice and glutinous rice to make porridge, and have in place of grains in your meals, as appropriate. For those with long-term deficiency and cold syndrome or diarrhea, add Chinese yam and gorgon fruit. TCM believes that japonica rice and glutinous rice have the effect of tonifying zhong qi, and strengthening the spleen and stomach; Chinese yam and gorgon fruit have the effect of strengthening the spleen and kidney, stabilizing astringency and stomach; glutinous rice is warm, which is also in line with the physiological characteristics of the stomach, preferring warm to cold. If making glutinous rice into snacks makes it too hard to digest for most people, then change the cooking method; making porridge with glutinous rice can help reap the benefits while avoiding the disadvantages, thereby achieving great results.

(2) Take 9 grams of Chinese yam, 9 grams of Liushenqu, 9 grams of millet sprouts, 9 grams of malt and 3 grams of licorice, and boil in water for 15 minutes. Turn off the heat, remove the dregs and then add rice to make porridge. It is a very effective and easy recipe for patients with stomach issues who often experience postprandial fullness. Chinese yam strengthens the spleen and nourishes the stomach, millet sprout and malt help with digestion and mediate the stomach; these three are the iron triangle for the protection of stomach qi. Liushenqu is sweet and warm and enters the stomach meridian, which is effective in dealing with indigestion and fullness of the stomach and abdomen; licorice tonifies and benefits zhong qi, eases urgency and

relieves pain. The combination of these can nourish the stomach and strengthen the spleen, thereby improving digestive function.

(3) Take 6 grams of oroxylum indicum and 9 grams of membrane of hen egg and cook with rice to make porridge. This is suitable for people with stomach pain on an empty stomach, which improves after eating, and for long-term care for patients with various types of gastric and duodenal mucosal erosions and ulcers. Oroxylum indicum is the dried mature seeds of *Oroxylum indicum* (L.) Vent, a plant of the family Bignoniaceae, which can detoxify the liver, harmonize the stomach and generate muscle. It can be used to treat stomach pain due to liver and stomach qi stagnation. Membrane of hen egg, commonly known as the inner membrane of the eggshell, is neutral and sweet in nature, enters the lung, spleen and stomach meridians, and has the effect of astringent exudation and promoting new tissue growth. These two drugs condition the liver qi, harmonize the stomach qi and promote the lung qi to protect the membrane and heal ulcers.

9. 喜闻乐见的"补药"真的适合你吗

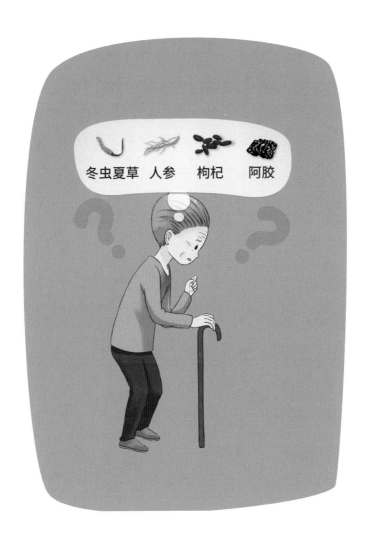

Q: 冬虫夏草价格昂贵，到底有用吗？

A: 我们一听到冬虫夏草四个字，第一反应就是名贵和大补。该药对于治疗肾阳亏虚、肺虚久咳、肾不纳气等证效果显著，且不易滋腻，无碍脾胃，从而成为逢年过节、走亲访友的馈赠佳品。

客观来说，冬虫夏草确实适用于肺肾两虚，尤其是偏肾阳虚的人，然而中医认为平衡是健康，阴平阳秘才是最好的身体状态，所以并不是每个人都需要吃补药，更不是每个人都需要补阳气，故服用冬虫夏草，还需要准确辨证。冬虫夏草之所以成为大众偏爱的补药，是因为其补力温和，不易补而瘀滞。但同时也意味着运用冬虫夏草滋补身体的时候，需要达到一定剂量才能取得预计的效果，一般要 20 ~ 30 g，依照目前的市场价格，大多数普通家庭会因此承担沉重的经济负担，还需量力而行。滋补肺肾的中药，并非只有冬虫夏草一种选择，而是百花齐放、各显神通，比如肺阴虚可以用百合，肺气涣散可以用蛤蚧粉，肾阴亏虚可以用枸杞子、桑椹，肾阳不足可以用鹿角胶和肉苁蓉等，同样可以起到不输冬虫夏草的作用，而价格则不足其百分之一。

Q：人参到底该怎么选？

A： 自古以来，人参一直都被奉为"补药之首"和"百草之王"。人参的药用价值极高，其几乎每个部位都有不可替代的作用，临床上最被推崇的作用就是补虚，具体应用以补气虚为主。然而不同品种的人参，其功效主治亦有不同，也就有了其各自对应的适用人群。

通常来说，人参分为三种：红参（高丽参）、西洋参（花旗参）和白参（生晒参）。红参性温，适合阳气不足、畏寒肢冷者；西洋参性凉，适合内热偏盛、口干乏力者；生晒参重在补气，无明显阴阳偏盛，单纯中气不足者更合适。

此外，重点说两个需要注意的问题，第一，并不是存在虚就一定适合用人参来滋补，如果兼有脾胃不足、湿邪偏盛，就暂时不适合服用人参，此类表现为脘腹胀满、周身困重、食欲不佳、大便黏腻，如果再服用人参，会助湿增邪，导致气血瘀滞，反而加重症状。需要在中医的诊治下先祛除湿气，再辨证进补。第二，野山参是上等的补气佳品，有挽大厦于倾倒之力，越来越多的人会不惜血本，在家中常备野山参。其实野山参虽然补力专宏，但是更适合极度虚弱者和耄耋老人，而非大多数人，掌握不好适应证，反而适得其反，况且野山参价格极高，真伪难辨，其实并不推荐作为居家补药储藏，相比而言，普通且价廉的生晒参虽然补力平和，但更适合常年服用，副作用也更小。

Q： 石斛究竟养胃吗？

A： 与人参、冬虫夏草等耳熟能详的补药不同，石斛这一味补药名气没那么大，但或许更加实用。经常可以听到患者问中医："石斛是不是养胃的啊？我能吃点石斛吗？"

中医认为"胃为阳明燥土，故喜润恶燥；脾为太阴湿土，故喜燥恶湿"，通俗地讲，胃喜欢滋润，脾喜欢干燥。石斛性微寒，入肺、胃、肾经，有滋阴、养胃、生津的功效，是一味不折不扣的具有滋润作用的补药。从这个角度来说，石斛确实有养胃的作用。

阴虚明显的胃病患者时常伴有口干、纳差、便秘、失眠等症状，石斛对于这类患者确实有着不错的养胃效果。但也有相当一部分脾胃虚寒或者寒滞肠胃的患者，表现为雷鸣腹痛、大便稀薄、喜温喜按、饮水或进食生冷后胃部不适，这个时候，石斛就不能服用了。另外，舌苔白或者厚腻的人，说明湿邪中阻，理应通阳化湿为先，具有滋阴作用的石斛也同样不合适。

Q: "保温杯泡枸杞"真的只是中年人的专利吗？

A: 时下形容一个中年人，都会用"保温杯泡枸杞"这个说法，其实，这正说明了一种社会现象，人们的工作和生活基本已经与电子产品深度捆绑，各种导致人们低头的电子屏幕霸占了几乎全部的碎片时间。长时间使用、观看电脑和手机，对眼睛的健康是非常有害的。视疲劳越来越低龄化的趋势已经不可阻挡，很多年轻人出现眼目干涩、视力下降、视物模糊等症状，而枸杞子正是我们眼睛的头号"保护神"。

枸杞子味甘性平，入肝、肾经，有补肾益精、养肝明目之功效。中医临床上常常运用枸杞子治疗肝肾亏虚引起的头晕目眩，效果很好。中药药理学研究显示，枸杞子富含的 β 胡萝卜素在人体内会转化成维生素A，后者可以生成视黄醇，从而提高视力。枸杞子还可以预防近视，消除眼疲劳，预防青光眼、干眼症以及白内障，这也是枸杞子特别适合中老年人和高度用眼者的理由所在。

目前市场上常见的枸杞子分为红枸杞和黑枸杞两种，后者还富含花青素，更偏重于抗氧化、抗衰老的作用。推荐使用红枸杞和黑枸杞以 1∶1 的比例，每日共 20 g，泡水喝。

另外，特别需要提醒的是，枸杞子是有一定甜度的药品，对于有烧心、反酸、嗳气等明显胃食管反流症状的患者来说，建议把浓度降低，并尽量保持水温温热，以减少增加反流的危险因素。

Q: 阿胶是女性的专属补药吗？

A: 在传统认知中，一说到阿胶，大家最常见的反应就是补血养颜、美容焕肤，所以阿胶自然而然地被打上了女性专属补品的标签，事实上，在中医理论中，阴不独长，阳不孤生，并没有哪一味药物是只有男性或者女性可以使用的，那么为什么阿胶在大众视野里就是女性所独享的呢？理由其实很简单，还是要从阿胶的功效与主治说起，阿胶为驴皮熬制的胶块，味甘，性微温，归肺、肝、肾经，有补血止血、滋阴润肺之功效，临床上用于治疗各种出血、贫血、月经不调、失眠烦躁。

阿胶首先是一味非常直接有效的补血药物。女性以血为先天，气血充盈，脉道通利，则面色红润，肤如凝脂，所以阿胶对于女性的养颜作用是毋庸置疑的。阿胶在调经方面也有着不可替代的作用，对于各种因气血亏虚引起的崩漏和经期异常，阿胶都是作为君药出现在处方中的。

那么男性到底能不能吃阿胶，什么情况下才适合吃阿胶呢？答案当然是肯定的，男性也有气血，也可能出现血虚伤阴，同样，男性如果有口干、烦躁失眠、面目无华、久咳无痰的症状，也应该使用阿胶来进行调补。就算是男性，也同样需要充足的精气神和容光满面的精神状态；就算是男性，也同样需要通过养血来实现"逆生长"。

关于阿胶这味补药，还有两个需要注意的地方，第一，阿胶乃血肉有情之品，又出自哺乳动物，饮片本身有着一定的腥气，在熬制阿胶的时候，需要用黄酒进行预制，建议浸泡12小时以上，并在隔水蒸的同时放入一定的生姜和红糖，或者冰糖以达到调整口味和去腥气的目的。阿胶性质厚腻，每日服用成膏不宜超过5 g。第二，当年出品的阿胶性温燥，即刻拿来入药易灼犯真阴，导致出现烦躁、上火等症状。阿胶主张越陈越好，性越平和，建议有用阿胶滋补习惯的人，定期购买储藏，取陈三年以上的阿胶收膏服用，可避免温热之嫌。

9. Are popular tonics the right choice for you

Q: Cordyceps sinensis is expensive; does it really work?

A: When we hear the words "Cordyceps sinensis", the first thought is that it is expensive and a great tonic. This medicine is effective in treating kidney yang deficiency, lung deficiency and persistent coughing, and kidney failure to receive qi. It does not over-nourish and does not hinder the spleen or stomach, which makes it a good gift for visiting friends and relatives during the holidays.

Objectively speaking, Cordyceps sinensis is suitable for people with deficiency in both lung and kidney, especially those leaning towards kidney yang deficiency. However, TCM believes that balance is health and dynamic equilibrium between yin and yang is best. So, not everyone needs to take tonics, and not everyone needs to supplement yang qi, so consuming Cordyceps sinensis also requires accurate syndrome differentiation. Cordyceps sinensis has become a popular tonic because of its mild tonic power, which will not easily lead to stagnation. However, it also means that when using Cordyceps sinensis to nourish the body, a certain dosage is needed to achieve the expected effect, usually 20–30 grams. Based on the current market price, most ordinary families will bear a heavy financial burden and must decide based on their economic conditions. Moreover, Cordyceps sinensis is not the only TCM that can nourish the lung and kidney; instead, there are many others, each with its own effect. For example, lily bulbs can be used for lung yin deficiency, tokay gecko powder can be used for lung qi laxity, barbary wolfberry fruit and mulberry fruit can be used for kidney yin deficiency, and deer-horn glue and desertliving cistanche can be used for kidney yang deficiency. All these can have similar effect of Cordyceps sinensis, at less than 1% of the price.

Q: *How exactly should I choose ginseng?*

A: Since ancient times, ginseng has been regarded as the "top tonic" and the "king of all herbs". Its medicinal value is so high that almost every one of its parts has an irreplaceable role. Its biggest clinical practice is to cure the deficiency, with specific applications mainly for qi deficiency. However, different varieties of ginseng have different efficacy and major functions, which gives each of them corresponding groups of people for whom they are suitable.

Generally speaking, there are three types of ginseng: red ginseng (Korean ginseng), American ginseng and white ginseng (dried fresh ginseng). Red ginseng is warm in nature and is suitable for those who suffer from yang deficiency and cold limbs. American ginseng is cool in nature and is suitable for those who suffer from internal heat, dryness, thirst and fatigue; the main function of dried fresh ginseng is nourishing qi, and it is more suitable for those who do not have clear yin or yang deficiency and are simply deficient in zhong qi.

In addition, there are two important things to note. Firstly, ginseng is not suitable for everyone with a deficiency. Those with spleen and stomach deficiency and dampness are not suitable for taking ginseng at this stage. Main manifestations include fullness, heaviness, poor appetite and sticky stool. Taking ginseng will lead to increased dampness and evil qi, as well as stagnation of qi and blood, which will aggravate the symptoms. It is necessary to remove dampness first with consultation and treatment from a TCM practitioner and then take tonic based on syndrome differentiation. Secondly, wild ginseng is a superior tonic, with the power to "save the building from collapsing", so an increasing number of people spare no expense and always have wild ginseng at home. In fact, although wild ginseng has a special tonic power, it is more suitable for the extremely weak and the elderly, not for most people. Else, it could actually do damage. Besides, it is extremely expensive, and it's hard to tell the real from the fake. So, it is not recommended to store wild ginseng at home as a tonic. Comparatively, the good and cheap dried fresh ginseng, while with only neutral tonic power, is suitable for long-term consumption and has fewer side effects.

Q: *Does dendrobium actually nourish the stomach?*

A: Different from familiar tonics such as ginseng and Cordyceps sinensis, this tonic is not very well-known but perhaps more practical. You can often hear patients asking TCM practitioners: "If dendrobium nourishes the stomach, can I have some dendrobium?"

TCM believes that "the stomach is yangming channel, so it prefers moisture to dryness, while the spleen is taiyin channel, so it prefers dryness to wetness". Simply put, the stomach likes to be moistened, and the spleen likes to be dry. From this point of view, dendrobium does have the effect of nourishing the stomach.

Patients with yin deficiency and gastric issues, often concomitant with dryness, thirst, poor appetite constipation, and insomnia. Dendrobium will play a positive role in nourishing the stomach for this type of person. However, there is also a considerable portion of patients with deficient cold spleen and stomach, whose manifestations are stomach growling, thin stools, preferring warmth and dampness, stomach discomfort after drinking water or eating raw or cold food. Dendrobium should not be taken in this condition. In addition, white or thick and greasy tongue coating indicates that dampness is blocked, so it is necessary to remove the blockage and alleviate the dampness first. Dendrobium, which has the effect of nourishing yin, is also inappropriate.

Q: *Drinking barbary wolfberry fruit in thermos cups, is it really only for the middle-aged person?*

A: Nowadays, to describe a middle-aged person, many will use the rhetoric of "barbary wolfberry fruit water in a thermos cup". In fact, this is to illustrate a social phenomenon where people's work and life have basically been deeply bound with electronic products, all kinds of electronic screens that lead people to get glued to the screen almost all the time. The prolonged use of computers and cellphones is very harmful to the eyes. Visual fatigue has been occurring among the younger population, and many young people are experiencing dry eyes, reduced vision and blurred vision, and barbary wolfberry fruit is the number one protector of the eyes.

Barbary wolfberry fruit is sweet and neutral, enters the liver and kidney meridians,and has the effect of tonifying the kidney, benefiting the essence, nourishing the liver and brightening the eyes. TCM often uses barbary wolfberry fruit clinically to treat vertigo and dimming caused by liver and kidney deficiency, with good results. Pharmacological studies in TCM have shown that the β-carotene rich in barbary wolfberry fruit is converted into vitamin A in the body, which produces retinol and thus improves vision. Barbary wolfberry fruit can also help prevent myopia, eliminate eye fatigue,and prevent glaucoma, dry eye disease and cataracts, which is the reason why barbary wolfberry fruit is particularly suitable for the elderly and those glued to electronics.

The most common barbary wolfberry fruit on the market today includes red barbary wolfberry fruit and black barbary wolfberry fruit. The latter also rich in anthocyanins and has better antioxidant and anti-aging effects. It is recommended to put equal part red and black barbary wolfberry fruit, a total of 20 grams per day in water to drink.

In addition, it is especially important to remember that barbary wolfberry fruit have a certain degree of sweetness, and for patients with heartburn, acid reflux, belching and other obvious GERD symptoms, it is recommended to reduce the concentration and try to keep the water warm to reduce the risk factors that increase reflux.

Q: *Is ass hide glue (Colla Corii Asini) a tonic exclusively for women?*

A: In the traditional perception, the most common reaction when it comes to ass hide glue is that it nourishes the blood and skin, so it is often naturally labeled as a women-only tonic, but in fact, in TCM theory, yin and yang cannot be separated. There is no medicine that can only be used for men or women, so why is ass hide glue exclusive to women in the public eye? The reason is actually simple, based on the efficacy and major function of ass hide glue. Ass hide glue is black gum boiled from donkey skin, which tastes sweet, has a slightly warm property, and is in the lung, liver, and kidney meridians. It can nourish the blood, stop bleeding, nourish yin and moisten the lungs. Clinically, it is used to treat bleeding, anemia, menstrual disorders, insomnia and irritability.

It is a very direct and effective blood tonic for women. Qi and blood are paramount for women. When they are abundant, and the veins are smooth, women's faces will be rosy, and the skin will be smooth and shiny, so there is no doubt that ass hide glue is good for women. Besides ass hide glue has an irreplaceable role in regulating menstruation and is found in prescriptions as the "Monarch" for all kinds of menorrhagia and menstrual abnormalities caused by deficiency of qi and blood.

So, can men take ass hide glue, and under what circumstances? The answer is of course yes, men also have qi and blood and may also have blood deficiency and injury to yin. Similarly, men who have dry mouth, irritability and insomnia, dullness, and cough without phlegm should also take ass hide glue to regulate the symptoms. Even men need sufficient qi and a great spirit; even men need to nourish their blood to "appear younger".

There are two other things to note about this tonic. Firstly, ass hide glue is an animal product from mammals, so the tablets have a certain fishy smell. When boiling ass hide glue, it is recommended to soak it in rice wine for more than 12 hours and add some ginger and brown sugar (or crystal sugar) when steaming to adjust the taste and remove the fishy smell. In addition, ass hide glue is thick and greasy in nature, so it is advisable to note take more than 5 grams per day and stick with it in the long haul. Secondly, the new ass hide glue produced this year is warm and dry. If immediately used in medicine, it can induce irritability and heatiness. For ass hide glue, the older, the better, becasue its nature will be more neutral. It is recommended that people who have the habit of taking ass hide glue regularly buy it to store at home and consume ass hide glue from more than three years ago to avoid warmth and heat.

10. 发现淋巴结肿大怎么办

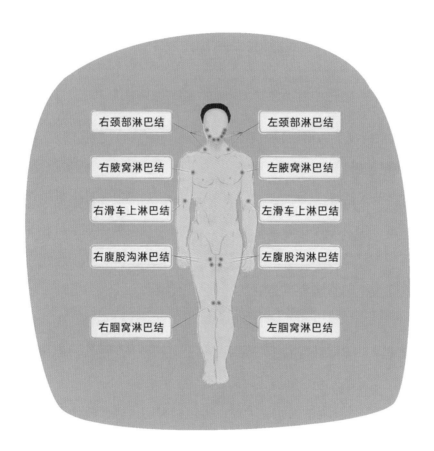

Q： 什么是淋巴结？

A： 淋巴结是人体淋巴器官的一种，是人体免疫系统的重要组成部分。（划重点：正常人都有淋巴结，不要一看到超声写的颈部可见小淋巴结就紧张得不能自已。）

淋巴结的主要功能：滤过淋巴液、产生淋巴细胞和进行免疫应答。简而言之，淋巴结可以帮助机体抵御外界致病因素。

淋巴结的分布：淋巴结多成群分布，按其在身体部位的深浅可分为深淋巴结和浅淋巴结。我们可触及到的淋巴结通常为浅淋巴结，多位于身体的颈部（包括锁骨上）、肘窝、腋窝、腹股沟、腘窝等处。

Q： 什么叫淋巴结肿大？在家如何进行淋巴结触诊？

A： 正常情况下，淋巴结直径 2 ～ 5 mm，不易触及；可触及到的淋巴结（如上文提到的浅淋巴结）质地柔软，表面光滑，推动时与周围组织没有粘连感。淋巴结肿大多为局限性（约 75%），其中超过 50% 的淋巴结肿大发生在头颈部。当某些器官或部位发生病变时，细菌、毒素、寄生虫或肿瘤细胞可在淋巴液中经淋巴管进入相应部位的淋巴结，该淋巴结进行阻截和清除，从而阻止病变扩散。此时淋巴结中发生细胞增殖等变化，导致淋巴结肿大。

进行淋巴结触诊可以帮助我们判断引起淋巴结肿大的原因，那我们在家如何监测淋巴结变化，如何进行淋巴结触诊呢？上文已经介绍了浅淋巴结的部位，触诊时需要关注位置、大小、质地、疼痛。

（1）位置：当发现淋巴结肿大时，可以同时通过触诊其他浅淋巴结区域进行局限性淋巴结肿大还是全身性淋巴结肿大的初步判断。触诊部位包括双侧颈部（含锁骨上）、腋窝、肘窝（滑车上）、腹股沟、腘窝。

（2）大小：临床医学触诊中常以淋巴结直径表示淋巴结大小，颈部和腋窝淋巴结直径 >1 cm 或锁骨上淋巴结直径 >0.5 cm 或腹股沟淋巴结直径 >1.5 cm 为异常肿大淋巴结。

（3）质地：一般认为，质地柔软、活动性极好的淋巴结，恶性的可能性相对小。

（4）疼痛：疼痛被认为与炎症相关，可能是急性感染导致淋巴结肿大的提示，恶性的可能性相对较小，但是对于伴有疼痛的快速、进行性增大的淋巴结，则需高度警惕为恶性肿大。

Q： 哪些疾病可能会引起淋巴结肿大？

A： 包括感染、自身免疫性疾病、恶性肿瘤和其他一些罕见情况。

（1）感染：多见于由引流区域的急、慢性炎症引起，如急性化脓性扁桃体炎、齿龈炎可引起颈部淋巴结肿大。会阴部感染时也可出现腹股沟淋巴结肿大。淋巴结肿大也可见于全身性感染性疾病，例如传染性单核细胞增多症、结核病、梅毒等。肿大的淋巴结多柔软，常有压痛，表面光滑、无粘连，肿大至一定程度即停止，多会随着炎症消退好转。

（2）自身免疫性疾病：多见于但不限于系统性红斑狼疮、干燥综合征、结节病、坏死性淋巴结炎等。

（3）恶性肿瘤：恶性肿瘤转移所致肿大的淋巴结，质地坚硬，或有橡皮样感，表面可光滑或突起，与周围组织粘连，不易推动，一般无压痛。胸部肿瘤如肺癌可向右侧锁骨上淋巴结转移；胃癌多向左侧锁骨上淋巴结转移。此外，急、慢性白血病，淋巴瘤，恶性组织细胞病等也常以淋巴结肿大为主要表现。

（4）其他：一些罕见原因，例如苯妥英钠等药物副作用。

Q： 淋巴结肿大是否提示恶性肿瘤？

A： 上文已经提到，出现淋巴结肿大的原因有很多。事实上，恶性肿瘤只占其中一小部分。一项荷兰的研究发现在 2556 例由家庭医生发现的淋巴结肿大的患者中，10% 由医生判断需要进行活检，只有 1.1% 的患者的淋巴结肿大与恶性肿瘤相关。美国的一项研究也发现，238 例淋巴结肿大的患者中，只有 3 例被证实肿大淋巴结与恶性肿瘤相关。因此，发现淋巴结肿大时过度的焦虑和紧张是不必要的。

Q: 什么情况下需要到医院就诊？

A: 一些肿大的淋巴结常常随着一定区域感染的好转而好转，有自愈倾向。但对于以下情况，应推荐到医院就诊。

（1）无明显诱因的淋巴结肿大。

（2）持续性肿大超过两周，或进行性增大。

（3）淋巴结质硬或活动度不佳。

（4）伴有全身症状，例如盗汗、发热、体重下降。

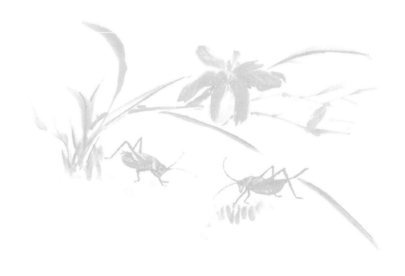

10.What should I do if I find my lymph nodes swollen

Q: What are lymph nodes?

A: Lymph nodes are a type of lymphatic organ in the human body and an important part of the immune system. (Emphasizing that everyone has lymph nodes. Don't get nervous just because you see "small nodes visible" on your ultrasound results.)

The main functions of lymph nodes are filtrating lymphatic fluid, producing lymphocytes and providing an immune response. In short, lymph nodes help the body defend itself against external pathogenic factors.

Distribution of lymph nodes: Lymph nodes are mostly distributed in groups and can be divided into deep and superficial ones based on their depth in the body parts. Lymph nodes we can palpate are usually superficial ones, mostly located in the neck (including collarbone), cubital fossa, armpit, groin and popliteal fossa.

Q: What do swollen lymph nodes mean? How to perform lymph node palpation at home?

A: Normally, lymph nodes are 2–5 mm in diameter and are not easily palpable; those that are palpable (such as the superficial lymph nodes mentioned above) are soft with a smooth surface, and do not feel adherent to the surrounding tissue when pushed. Swollen lymph nodes are mostly (about 75%) local, with more than 50% occurring in the neck. When lesions occur in certain organs or areas, bacteria, toxins, parasites or tumor cells in the lymphatic fluid can enter the lymph nodes in the corresponding areas via the lymphatic vessels. The lymph nodes can block and remove them, thus stopping the spread of the lesions. At this time, cell proliferation and other changes occur in the lymph nodes, resulting in them being swollen.

Performing lymph node palpation can help us determine the cause of swollen lymph nodes. So, how do we monitor lymph node changes at home and perform lymph node palpation? The site of the superficial lymph nodes has been described above. When palpating, pay attention to the location, size, texture and pain.

(1) Location: When you find swollen lymph nodes, palpate other superficial lymph node areas to initially determine whether the swelling is local or generalized. Palpation sites include both sides of the neck (including collarbone), armpit, cubital fossa (epitrochlea), groin and popliteal fossa.

(2) Size: The size of a lymph node is often indicated by diameter in clinical palpation. Cervical and axillary lymph nodes >1 cm, supraclavicular lymph nodes >0.5 cm or inguinal lymph nodes >1.5 cm are considered abnormal and swollen lymph nodes.

(3) Texture: It is generally believed that if the lymph nodes are soft and extremely mobile, the likelihood of malignancy is relatively low.

(4) Pain: Pain is thought to be associated with inflammation and may indicate that the swelling is caused by acute infection, with relatively low likelihood of malignancy. However, one should be highly alert to the rapid and progressive growing

of lymph nodes with pain, as it may be malignant.

Q: *What diseases may cause swollen lymph nodes?*

A: Infections, autoimmune diseases, malignant tumor and some other rare conditions.

(1) Infection: Swollen lymph nodes are most often caused by acute and chronic inflammation in the lymphatic drainage areas. For example, acute purulent tonsillitis and gingivitis can cause swollen lymph nodes in the neck. Perineal infection may also cause swollen inguinal lymph nodes. Swollen lymph nodes can also be due to systemic infectious diseases such as infectious mononucleosis, tuberculosis and syphilis. In most cases, swollen lymph nodes are soft, often with pressure pain; they have a smooth surface and no adhesions. The lymph nodes will stop growing at a certain level and get better as the inflammation subsides.

(2) Autoimmune diseases: Mostly seen in but not limited to systemic lupus erythematosus, Sjögren syndrome, thyroid nodules, and necrotizing lymphadenitis.

(3) Malignant tumor: Swollen lymph nodes due to malignant tumor metastasis are hard or rubbery in texture, with smooth or raised surfaces. They adhere to surrounding tissues, and are not easily pushed, generally without pressure pain. Thoracic tumors such as lung cancer can metastasize to the right supraclavicular lymph nodes; stomach cancer mostly metastasizes to the left supraclavicular lymph nodes. In addition, acute and chronic leukemia, lymphoma, and malignant histiocytosis are often manifested by swollen lymph nodes.

(4) Others: Some rare causes, such as side effects of drugs like phenytoin.

Q: Do swollen lymph nodes indicate malignant tumors?

A: As mentioned above, swollen lymph nodes can be caused by many factors. In fact, malignant tumors account for only a small percentage of them. A Dutch study found that of 2556 patients with swollen lymph nodes detected by their family physician, 10% required a biopsy according to the physician, and only 1.1% were associated with malignant tumors. Data from a study in the United States also found that of 238 patients with swollen lymph nodes, only 3 were confirmed to be associated with malignant tumors. Therefore, don't stress too much if you find swollen lymph nodes.

Q: When do I need to go to the hospital?

A: Swollen lymph nodes often get better as local infections subside and heal on their own. However, a hospital visit is recommended for the following cases.

(1) Swollen lymph nodes with no clear cause.

(2) Lymph nodes constantly swollen for more than two weeks, or have grown progressively.

(3) Lymph nodes are hard or have poor mobility.

(4) Swollen lymph nodes accompanying systemic symptoms, such as night sweats, fever, and weight loss.

11、心肺功能锻炼

面对病毒，靠什么活下来？靠的是人体的免疫和心肺功能。人体通过肺吸入充足的氧气，心脏要有充足的力量把氧气通过血液循环运送到全身。因此居家生活期间日常进行心肺功能锻炼显得尤为重要。

Q：什么是心肺功能锻炼？

A： 心肺功能是指人体将摄入的氧气转化为能量的能力，主要包括肺部摄氧能力、心脏通过泵血输送氧气至全身的效率，以及肌肉利用氧气的能力。肺的容量大小及活动次数直接影响氧气的摄取量，心脏跳动的强弱直接影响血液循环的效率。心肺功能表现出来就是人体能够承受运动负荷的耐受能力。

心肺功能锻炼是指通过一定的锻炼提高人体肺通气、心脏泵血和肌肉组织利用氧气的能力。进行心肺功能锻炼一方面可以改善血液循环，促进血液流动，另一方面有助于增强心肌的收缩能力，提高每搏心输出量。

Q：哪些人适合心肺功能锻炼？

A： 心肺功能不佳的表现主要有以下几点：①运动吃力，特别是爬楼梯、跑步、跑跳时出现胸闷、气喘。②日常呼吸困难、头晕、心慌、胸痛、颈静脉怒张、双下肢水肿等。

居家生活的人都适合进行心肺功能锻炼，以提高免疫力。患有肺心病、高血压、心力衰竭、心功能不全、慢性阻塞性肺疾病等疾病的人尤其要注重日常心肺功能锻炼。

Q： 居家生活期间心肺功能锻炼有哪些方式？

A： 心肺功能锻炼最简单的办法是有氧运动，每周进行 3～4 次中等强度的运动，能够在很大程度上提高心肺功能。居家生活期间心肺功能锻炼的方式如下。

（1）练习深呼吸锻炼肺部的收缩能力：深度吸气，让气体在肺部停留几秒，然后再深度呼出。

（2）跳绳：加快呼吸和心率，有利于血液获得更多的氧气，增强心肺功能。

（3）练太极拳：太极拳讲究腹式呼吸，可加大肺部的容气量，还可以舒张血管，改善血液循环。

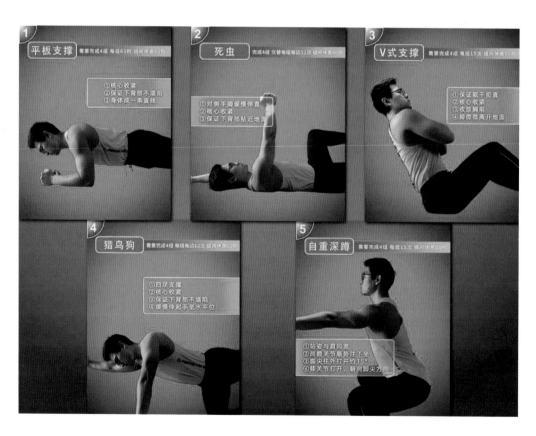

（4）借助健身器械如哑铃、跑步机等锻炼，可增加胸腔的容量和心脏收缩力。

（5）下蹲运动，锻炼大腿肌肉，对提高心肺功能有明显作用。

（6）注意良好的生活状态，保持心情舒畅，也会促进心肺功能的改善。

我们团队联合江江教练，推出了一套可行性高、科学性强的居家锻炼动作。

Q: 不同人群如何选择心肺功能锻炼的类型？

A: 年轻人可选择跳绳或健身器械辅助锻炼，中等强度，可以用心率来反映，相当于靶心率＝（220－年龄）×（60%～80%），每次运动 20～60 分钟，每周 5～6 次。

中老年人可以选择练习太极拳、健身气功如八段锦等。每天练习 40 分钟左右，动作与呼吸协调配合，以达到"气沉丹田"的效果。研究发现，长期练习太极拳能增大肺活量，还能改善神经调节、内分泌等全身功能。练习八段锦可以使膈肌上下运动大幅度增加，长期练习可以增大肺活量，显著改善呼吸耐力。

对于慢性肺源性心脏病合并心力衰竭的患者，病情稳定时，可练习深呼吸或吹气球，使气球直径达到 10～30 cm，每次 5～10 分钟，每天 3 次。

11.Cardiopulmonary exercises

What helps us survive in the face of viruses? It is immunity and cardiopulmonary fitness. We need to inhale sufficient oxygen through the lung, and the heart needs to have sufficient power to transport oxygen through the blood circulation to the whole body. This makes daily cardiopulmonary exercises especially important when staying at home.

Q: *What is cardiopulmonary exercise?*

A: Cardiopulmonary function refers to the body's ability to convert inhaled oxygen into energy, mainly including the ability of the lung to take in oxygen, the efficiency of the heart to transport oxygen to the whole body by pumping blood, and the ability of the muscles to utilize oxygen. The capacity of the lung and repository rate directly affect oxygen intake, and the strength of the heartbeat directly affects the efficiency of blood circulation. Cardiopulmonary function is the ability of the body to withstand exercise loads.

Cardiopulmonary exercises refer to certain exercises that can improve the body's ability to ventilate through the lung, pump blood to the heart and use oxygen in muscle tissues. Cardiopulmonary exercises can improve blood circulation and blood flow, improve the contraction capacity of the heart muscle, and increase cardiac output per beat.

Q: *Cardiopulmonary exercises are for what type of people?*

A: The main signs of poor cardiopulmonary function are as follows: ① Exercising feels strenuous, especially having chest tightness and shortness of breath when climbing stairs, running or jumping. ② Difficulty breathing in everyday life, dizziness, palpitation, chest pain, jugular vein distention, and lower limb edema.

Cardiopulmonary exercises are appropriate for anyone when staying at home to improve immunity. People suffering from pulmonary heart disease, hypertension, heart failure, cardiac insufficiency, chronic obstructive pulmonary disease and other diseases should pay special attention to daily cardiopulmonary exercises.

Q: *What are some types of cardiopulmonary exercises when staying at home?*

A: The easiest way is aerobic exercise. 3–4 times a week of moderate intensity exercise can improve cardiopulmonary function greatly. Some cardiopulmonary exercises when staying at home are as follows.

(1) Practicing deep breathing to exercise the contraction of the lung. Inhale deeply, hold the breath in the lung for a few seconds, and then exhale deeply.

(2) Jumping rope: It can speed up breathing and heart rate, help blood get more oxygen and improve cardiopulmonary function.

(3) Practice Tai Chi. Tai Chi emphasizes abdominal breathing, which can increase the capacity of the lung and widen the blood vessels to improve blood circulation.

(4) Exercise using fitness equipment such as dumbbells and treadmills can

increase chest cavity and heart contraction capacity.

(5) Squatting exercises, which exercise the thigh muscles, have a significant effect on improving cardiopulmonary function.

(6) Maintaining a healthy lifestyle and a relaxed mood will also promote improved cardiopulmonary function.

Our team, with Coach Jiangjiang, has introduced a set of highly feasible and scientific at-home exercises.

Q: *How do I choose the type of cardiopulmonary exercises?*

A: Young people can choose jumping rope or exercises with fitness equipment. The moderate intensity can be reflected by heart rate, equivalent to target heart rate = (220−age) × (60% to 80%). Each workout should last for 20–60 minutes, for 5–6 workouts per week.

Middle-aged and elderly people can choose Tai Chi, and fitness Qigong such as Baduanjin. Practice for about 40 minutes daily, with coordinated movements and breathing, to achieve Dantian breathing. Studies have found that long-term Tai Chi practice can increase lung capacity and improve neuromodulation, endocrine and other systemic functions. Baduanjin exercise can significantly increase diaphragm movement, and long-term practice can increase lung capacity and respiratory endurance.

For patients with chronic pulmonary heart disease concomitant with heart failure, when the condition is stable, you can practice deep breathing, or blowing balloons up to 10–30 cm in diameter for 5–10 minutes each time, 3 times a day.

12、静脉血栓·小·问答

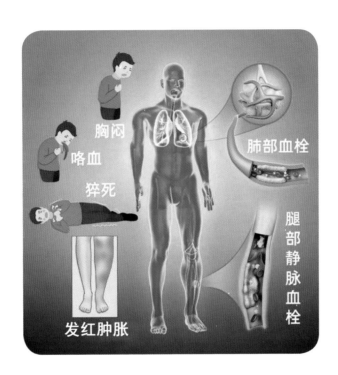

Q: 什么是静脉血栓？

A: "静脉血栓"是一个医学用语，多指血液在静脉腔内不正常凝结所形成的血凝块（栓子）。最常见的静脉血栓类型是腿部的深静脉血栓（DVT）。国外数据显示每年1000个成年人中就有1～3人受到静脉血栓的影响。DVT患者经常同时存在多种引起血栓形成的危险因素。但是在某些人群中，静脉血栓与基因缺陷相关，而没有静脉血栓形成的明显原因。

当血凝块在静脉中形成后，血液不能正常流过。久而久之，由于血流淤滞，阻塞处周围组织水肿并可伴有疼痛表现。在静脉血栓形成的早期阶段，主要风险是血凝块可能会进一步增大，或者血凝块发生移动并转移到肺部引起肺栓塞。肺栓塞是一种非常危险的疾病，据统计 10% 的肺栓塞患者因没有及时治疗而死亡。

Q： 为什么会出现静脉血栓？

A： 静脉血栓的病因因人而异。通常静脉中出现血凝块是由一个或多个因素导致：①静脉血流减慢；②静脉壁受损；③血流黏稠度增加。

一些特定情况可以增加血凝块形成的风险，常见原因包括年龄的增长、长期卧床或活动量下降、近期的手术或住院、肿瘤、怀孕、使用某些种类的口服避孕药或激素替代疗法、肥胖以及长距离旅行等。居家生活减少了人们的日常活动，久坐不动的时间更长，也会增加静脉血栓形成的风险。

Q： 静脉血栓的症状是什么？

A： 下肢 DVT 通常表现为小腿疼痛、发红并伴有肿胀，有肌肉紧张、收缩，不能自然伸开。有时 DVT 的症状会影响到整个腿部，特别是血栓较为广泛且影响到腹部静脉时。然而个体表现略有不同，并且在某些情况下可能没有明显的表现或体征，特别是血凝块仅出现在小腿部肌间静脉丛中时。上肢的 DVT 可以表现为肿胀、疼痛和发热，也可以表现为皮肤发蓝或发白。

肺栓塞症状多样，多表现为不明原因的活动后呼吸困难及气促、胸痛、咯血、烦躁不安、惊恐、濒死感甚至晕厥。肺栓塞三联征包括呼吸困难、胸痛及咯血，但仅有 20% 的患者会出现这种典型表现。

当下肢浅静脉血栓（SVT）形成时，通常表现为腿部有一条变硬、增厚、发红和疼痛的浅静脉。受到炎症影响，静脉的表面皮肤会发暗。发生 SVT 的患者通常有静脉曲张病史。

Q： 如何在居家生活中预防静脉血栓形成？

A： 需要做到以下四点。

（1）保持良好的生活习惯。多喝水，控制好血糖、血压、血脂，并且戒烟、戒酒。

（2）缩短久坐不动的时间，保持规律运动。每坐 1 小时左右起身活动一下，可以做下蹲动作或脚踝的屈伸动作，促进下肢血液循环，也可以适当抬高下肢，促进静脉回流。

（3）卧床患者注意定时变换体位，可以尝试做一下床上活动，如脚踝屈伸与环转运动、膝盖伸缩运动等。

（4）发现肿胀、疼痛、皮肤温度和色泽变化及感觉异常等，应及时就医。

12. Q&A on venous thromboembolism

Q: What is venous thromboembolism (VTE)?

A: VTE is a medical term for a blood clot (embolus) that forms when blood clots abnormally in the lumen of a vein. The most common type of VTE is deep vein thrombosis (DVT) in the legs. Based on data from other countries, 1–3 out of 1000 adults are affected by VTE every year. Patients with DVT often have multiple coexisting risk factors for thrombosis. However, in some populations, VTE are associated with genetic defects without a clear cause of VTE.

When a blood clot forms in a vein, blood cannot flow through it properly. Over time, the blockage of blood flow leads to edema and pain in the tissues surrounding the obstruction. In the early stages of VTE, the main risk is that the blood clots may continue to grow or that the blood clots may move and travel to the lung, causing a pulmonary embolism (PE). PE is a very dangerous disease; it is estimated that 10% of patients with PE die due to lack of timely treatment.

Q: Why does VTE occur?

A: The cause of VTE varies depending on the individual. The presence of blood clots in vein is usually caused by one or more of the following factors: ① slowing of venous blood flow; ② damage to the venous wall; ③ increased blood viscosity.

A number of specific conditions can increase the risk of blood clots formation.

Common causes include increasing age, prolonged bed rest or decreased activity, recent surgery or hospitalization, tumors, pregnancy, use of certain types of oral contraceptives or hormone replacement therapy, obesity, and long-distance travel. Staying at home reduces the number of daily activities and increases the risk of VTE due to being sedentary for long periods of time.

Q: *What are the symptoms of VTE?*

A: DVT in the legs usually manifests as a painful, red and swollen calf, with muscle tension, contraction and inability to stretch naturally. Sometimes the symptoms of DVT can affect the entire leg, especially blood clots are more extensive and affect the abdominal veins. However, manifestations on individuals vary slightly. In some cases, there may not be obvious manifestations or signs, especially if the blood clots are present only in the intramuscular venous plexus of the calf. DVT in the upper limbs can manifest as swelling, pain, fever, or as bluish or pale skin.

PE has a variety of symptoms, mostly unexplained dyspnea and shortness of breath after activity, chest pain, hemoptysis, irritability, panic, a sense of impending doom and even syncope. The PE triad includes dyspnea, chest pain, and hemoptysis, but only 20% of the patients will have these typical symptoms.

When a superficial vein thrombosis (SVT) forms in a lower limb, it usually manifests as a hardened, thickened, red and painful superficial vein in the leg. The skin on the surface of the vein is darkened by inflammation. Patients who develop SVT usually have a history of varicose veins.

Q: How can I prevent VTE when staying at home?

A: Pay attention to the following points.

(1) Maintain a healthy lifestyle. Drink more water, control blood sugar, blood pressure and cholesterol, and quit smoking and drinking.

(2) Reduce sedentary time and exercise regularly. Get up and move around every hour or so. You can do squats or ankle flexion and extension movements to promote blood circulation in the lower limbs. Elevating the lower limbs can also promote venous return.

(3) Bedridden patients should change their position regularly and try to do some exercises in bed, such as ankle flexion, extension and rotation, and knee stretching.

(4) If you find swelling, pain, changes in skin temperature and color and abnormal sensation, promptly seek medical attention.

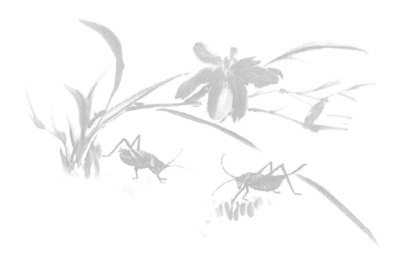

13、肿瘤化疗患者营养支持小问答

肿瘤患者营养不良发生率高，营养不良不仅影响患者的生活质量，也在一定程度上影响患者的临床结局。化疗药物大都会导致不同程度的胃肠道相关不良事件，从而导致营养不良的发生，故预防和治疗肿瘤化疗患者营养不良、提高患者生活质量和治疗耐受性至关重要。

Q： 什么是营养不良？

A： 营养不良是指能量、蛋白质和（或）其他营养素缺乏、过剩或失衡，导致对人体的形态（体型、体格和机体组成）、功能产生的可以观察到的不良影响的一种状态。在肿瘤患者中，肿瘤本身（例如消化道肿瘤患者的消化道机械性梗阻及消化吸收障碍、头颈及食管肿瘤患者的吞咽困难）和肿瘤治疗（例如化疗导致的恶心、纳差、呕吐，化疗及放疗导致的味觉异常，部分镇痛药物带来的肠蠕动减慢）均可能促使营养不良的发生和发展。

Q： 如何纠正肿瘤患者营养不良？

A： 合理有效的营养支持。营养支持主要由补充、支持和治疗三部分构成，其内容包括饮食指导、改善摄食、口服营养补充及人工营养支持（即肠内营养和肠外营养治疗）。通过上述方法供给机体适当的营养，减轻患者代谢紊乱和骨骼肌消耗，改善生理及免疫功能，缓解疲劳、厌食等症状，改善患者生活质量。

Q: 居家生活期间如何了解肿瘤患者对能量和营养的每日需求？（吃多少？吃什么？要不要去医院输营养液？）

A: 各国营养学会在相关指南中均指出，对于存在营养不良或营养风险的肿瘤患者，如果经口进食无法满足机体营养需求，只要患者肠道功能正常，首先推荐通过强化营养咨询来增加经口进食，即尽可能经口进食进行营养支持，在无法经口进食或经口进食无法满足机体营养需求时（即不能满足 60% 目标能量需要量超过 3 天），优先考虑鼻胃管或鼻肠管喂养。

（1）对患者的体重进行估计。

标准体重：身高 (cm) － 105。正常体重范围：标准体重 ±10%。

超重：超过标准体重 10%。

消瘦：低于标准体重 10%。

（2）肿瘤患者的目标能量需要量估计。

卧床患者：标准体重（kg）×（20 ～ 25）kcal。

有活动能力者：标准体重（kg）×（25 ～ 30）kcal。

超重者：在基础能量上减少 5 kcal/kg。

消瘦者：在基础能量上增加 5 kcal/kg。

让我们来举个例：

男性，55 岁，可下床活动，身高 178 cm，体重 70 kg。

估计标准体重为 73 kg，该患者的体重在正常体重范围内。

合理的能量摄入量为 73×（25 ～ 30)=1825 ～ 2190（kcal）。

（3）肿瘤患者的蛋白质需要量估计为每天 1.0 ～ 2.0 g/kg，对于老年、肿瘤不活动和合并全身性炎症的肿瘤患者，目标蛋白质需要量为每天 1.2 ～ 1.5 g/kg；急性或慢性肾功能不全的患者目标蛋白质需要量为每天 0.8 ～ 1.2 g/kg。

建议优质蛋白质占 30% ～ 50%。常见的优质蛋白质包括畜肉、禽肉、鱼类、虾类、蛋类、奶制品、大豆制品等。对于这类食物要注意平衡，因为富含蛋白质的同时，它们相对其他食物来说脂肪含量也较高，部分肿瘤患者因肿瘤及治疗的影响，对油脂类食物耐受性差，此时烹调方式应选择清炒、清蒸、水煮、炖等。

Q： 居家生活期间肿瘤患者对能量的摄入有何推荐？（怎么吃？）

A： 居家生活期间无专业人员指导的情况下，常常因缺乏食物称量工具，对于能量的估算误差较大，居家生活期间如何估算患者的能量摄入量？在这里推荐简单易行的食物手掌法，即一种通过变换手掌的形状来表示各种食物的量，从而快速评估能量摄入量的方法，如用一拳头表示主食和水果、用一捧或一把表示蔬菜、用一掌心表示荤菜。

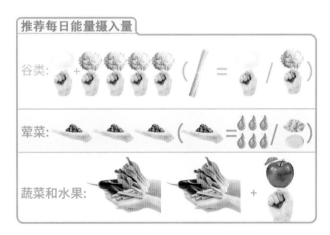

推荐的每日能量摄入量如下。

（1）谷类：一天一拳头馒头，四拳头米饭（一扎面条等于一拳头米饭或一拳头馒头）。

（2）荤菜：一天两或三掌心荤菜；一掌心荤菜约等于六只虾或一个鸡蛋大小的肉丝。

（3）蔬菜和水果：一天两捧蔬菜，深颜色蔬菜占一半；一拳头大小的水果。

Q: 居家生活期间化疗后骨髓抑制患者的饮食有哪些要求？

A: 化疗后患者常常出现白细胞及中性粒细胞减少，这些患者免疫力低下，感染风险较普通患者增高，因此在挑选及准备食物过程中对卫生要求较高。建议在准备处理食物前用热肥皂水清洗双手，处理生肉、家禽和海鲜前后应洗手；菜刀、砧板切配需生熟分开、荤素分开；菜刀、砧板、碗盘筷、厨房用布等在使用前和使用后应用热肥皂水或者杀菌消毒液彻底清洗。

所有食物应煮熟煮透，应避免吃溏心蛋、半熟牛肉、发芽土豆，查看食物有效期，切勿购买外包装有损坏或过期的食物，不饮用自己榨的蔬果汁，可考虑选择经过巴氏消毒并且密封包装完好的果汁。不购买卤菜、凉菜等熟食和路边摊食物，生肉、鱼虾等用包装袋分开包装，以免污染其他食物。

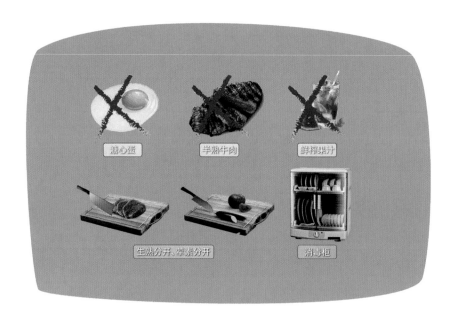

13. Q&A about nutrition support for chemotherapy patients

The incidence of malnutrition in tumor patients is high, and malnutrition not only affects patients' quality of life, but also influences the clinical outcome to some extent. Most chemotherapeutic drugs cause different degrees of gastrointestinal (GI)–related adverse events, which lead to malnutrition. Therefore, it is crucial to prevent and treat malnutrition in chemotherapy patients to improve their quality of life and treatment tolerance.

Q: What is malnutrition?

A: Malnutrition is a state in which a deficiency, excess or imbalance of energy, protein and/or other nutrients results in observable adverse effects on the body's morphology (build, physique and composition) and function. In tumor patients, both the tumor itself (e.g., mechanical obstruction of the GI tract and impaired digestion and absorption in GI tumor patients, dysphagia in neck and esophageal tumor patients) and the treatment (e.g., nausea, poor appetite and vomiting due to chemotherapy, dysgeusia due to chemotherapy and radiotherapy, and slowed bowel movement due to some pain medications) may contribute to the development and progression of malnutrition in tumor patients.

Q: How to correct malnutrition in tumor patients?

A: Through reasonable and effective nutritional support. Nutritional support mainly consists of three parts: supplementation, support and treatment, which include dietary guidance, improved feeding, oral nutritional supplementation and artificial nutritional support (i.e., enteral and parenteral nutrition therapy). These methods can supply the body with appropriate nutrition, reduce metabolic disorders and skeletal muscle depletion, improve physiological and immune functions, combat fatigue, anorexia and other symptoms, and improve the patient's quality of life.

> **Q:** How do I know the daily energy and nutritional requirements of tumor patients staying at home?(How much to eat? What to eat? Should I go to the hospital for nutrient supplementation solutions?)

A: National nutrition societies in various countries have pointed out in their guidelines that for tumor patients with malnutrition or nutritional risk, if oral feeding cannot meet the nutritional needs of the body, as long as the patient has a normal intestinal function, the first recommendation is to increase oral feeding through intensive nutritional counseling. That is, provide nutritional support through oral feeding as much as possible, and when oral feeding is not possible or when it cannot meet the nutritional needs (i.e., 60% of the target energy requirements cannot be met for more than 3 days), consider nasogastric tube or nasogastric tube feeding.

(1) Estimate the patients' weight.

Standard weight: height (cm) － 105. Normal weight range: standard weight

± 10%.

Overweight: > 110% standard weight.

Underweight: < 90% standard weight.

(2) Estimated target energy requirements for tumor patients.

Bedridden patients: standard weight (kg) × (20–25) kcal.

Mobile patients: Standard weight (kg) × (25–30) kcal.

Overweight: 5 kcal/kg reduction from basal energy.

Wasting: 5 kcal/kg increase on top of basal energy.

Here is an example.

For a 55–year–old male who is not bedridden, with a height of 178 cm and weight of 70 kg.

The estimated standard weight is 73 kg. So, his weight is within the normal range.

A moderate energy intake is 73 × (25–30) = 1825–2190 (kcal).

(3) Estimated protein requirements for tumor patients:1.0–2.0 g/kg per day. For the elderly, those with inactive tumor or with concomitant systemic inflammation, the target protein requirement is 1.2–1.5 g/kg per day; the target protein requirement for patients with acute or chronic renal insufficiency is 0.8–1.2 g/kg per day.

30%–50% of high–quality protein is recommended. Common high–quality proteins include livestock, poultry, fish, shrimp, eggs, dairy products, and soybean products. These foods need to be consumed in balance because while they are high in protein, they are also higher in fat than other foods. Some tumor patients have a low tolerance for high–fat foods due to tumor and treatment, hence stir–frying without oil, steaming, boiling and stewing are proper ways to prepare.

Q: What are the recommendations for energy intake for tumor patients when staying at home?(how to eat?)

A: Without professional guidance at home, calorie estimation is often inaccurate due to a lack of tools to weigh food. Here we recommend the simple and easy "palm method", a method to quickly assess food intake by changing the shape of your hand to indicate the amount of each food type. For example, a fist of grains and fruits, a handful of vegetables, and a palm size serving of meat.

The recommended daily intake is as follows.

(1) Grains: one fist of bun and four fists of rice per day (one fist of bun or rice equivalent of a serving of noodles).

(2) Meat dishes: two or three palm size servings of meat per day; one palm of meat dish is equal to about six shrimps or an egg–sized serving of shredded meat.

(3) Vegetables and fruits: two handfuls of vegetables, with half of them dark–colored, and one fist–sized piece of fruits per day.

Q: What are the dietary requirements for patients with myelosuppression after chemotherapy while staying at home?

A: Post–chemotherapy patients often have reduced white blood cells and neutrophils. They are immunocompromised and have a higher risk of infection than the average patient, and therefore require better hygiene during the selection and preparation of food. Wash your hands with warm soapy water before handling food, and before and after handling raw meat, poultry and seafood. Use different kitchen knives and cutting boards for raw and cooked meat and vegetables. Kitchen knives, cutting boards, bowls, dishes, chopsticks and washcloth should be thoroughly washed with warm soapy water or germicidal disinfectant before and after use.

All food should be cooked thoroughly; avoid eating soft−boiled eggs, half−cooked beef and sprouted potatoes. Check the expiration date of food; do not purchase food with damaged packaging or expired. Do not drink self−squeezed fruit and vegetable juices, consider choosing juice that is pasteurized with well−sealed packaging. Do not buy braised or cold dishes and other cooked or street food. Raw meat, fish and shrimps should be packed in separate bags to avoid cross−contamination.

14、心理问题如何疏导

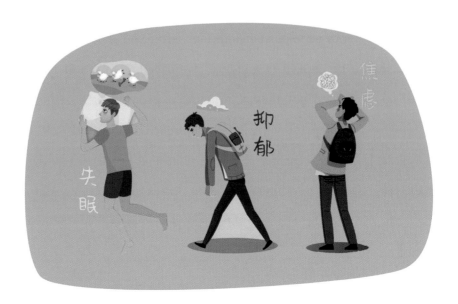

　　居家生活期间的节律容易紊乱，与人交流减少，工作线上沟通后出现较少的互动，容易出现情绪问题，比如抑郁情绪、焦虑情绪和睡眠问题。那么出现这类问题该如何应对呢？

Q: 我不开心，抑郁了怎么办？

A: 居家生活时要顺其自然、积极面对，不要预期将来。要坦然接受生活中发生的一切改变，认为这是生活的一部分，每一个环节都有惊喜的事情发生；不要把每一件不好的事情灾难化，即使是困难也要看到不开心总会过去。学会在不开心的经历中寻找一些乐趣，比如可以安排时间欣赏平时没有机会看的电影、玩游戏或阅读自己喜欢的书籍，寻找生活中积极的因素。

居家生活期间，定时起床和睡眠，定时运动和交流，让自己生活在一定的结构性生活中，有利于保持自己的生活节奏。多为家人做些事情，感受自己在家庭生活中的价值。要定期与家人交流，不要回避社交。

但是，如果情绪仍然非常低落，难以维持最基本的生活，则要寻找专业精神心理医生进行咨询。

Q: 我焦虑了怎么办？

A: 在居家生活中，一旦遇到自己无法预期的事件，就容易出现焦虑情绪，对将来过度担心、紧张。在干预这个情绪的过程中，不要过度预期将来，更不要灾难化地预期不好的结果。任何时候，都要告诉自己"总会有办法"。尤其当自己非常紧张，甚至出现躯体焦虑症状，如心慌、胸闷、出汗等时，不要惊慌，适当地深呼吸，播放一些钢琴轻音乐，让自己的注意力集中在外界事物，动手做一些简单的美食，做简单的家务，避免将注意力放在自己身上。如果非常紧迫，可以到医院进行一些基本的检查，在排除躯体疾病的情况下，在精神心理医生的帮助下服用一些苯二氮䓬类药物改善焦虑情绪。

Q: 我失眠了怎么办？

A: 居家生活非常容易昼夜节律紊乱，如果白天睡眠时间过长，容易出现夜间入睡困难。抑郁焦虑情绪突出时，容易出现失眠、入睡困难或者早醒。

因此，在出现睡眠困难时，一定要评估抑郁焦虑情绪，这个症状可能是抑郁焦虑情绪的一部分，对它们进行完整的评估，有利于早期更加全面地干预治疗。

　　失眠可能因为抑郁焦虑情绪所致。环境突然改变、过量饮用咖啡或者饮酒等因素，亦可导致入睡困难、早醒或夜间睡眠质量差，进而白天仍然感觉困倦，学习、工作难以集中注意力，出现情绪不稳定或者社交功能受到影响。

　　居家生活期间，如果持续出现睡眠问题，可以连续记录自己的上床时间、入睡时间、夜间醒来次数、总睡眠时长、早醒次数、白天的情绪和工作能力状况，用来辅助评估自己的情绪和睡眠状况。

　　如果出现睡眠问题，要放松心情，不要夸大睡眠带来的问题，尽量避免因为晚上睡眠困难而白天补偿性睡眠，尽量保持白天按照原来的节奏工作、生活。

　　晚上避免进行过分激烈的运动，避免听激烈的音乐和看恐怖的电影，避免过多时间看手机，让自己在安静的状态下入眠。可以睡前看一会书，避免过早躺在床上等待睡眠，上床睡觉时不预期睡眠带来的影响，坦然接受所有的睡眠状况。如果持续睡眠困难，可以到精神心理科就诊，配用少量的助眠药物。

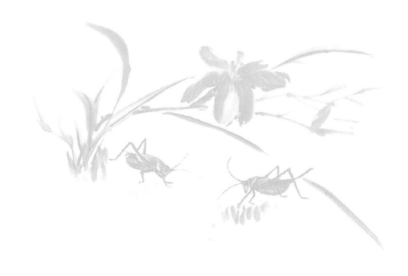

14. How to manage mental health

When staying at home, the rhythm of life tends to be disrupted. Less communication with people, and less interaction after online meetings make it more likely to develop issues of emotional health, such as depression, anxiety and trouble sleeping. So, how to deal with this type of issue?

Q: *What should I do if I am unhappy or depressed?*

A: When staying at home, you should let nature take its course and face it with positivity and without anticipating the future. Be open to all the changes that happen in life and consider it a part of life. Surprises can occur anytime, so try not to see every bad thing as a catastrophe; even if it is difficult to comprehend, unhappiness will always pass, and it is just a part of life. Learn to find something fun within the unpleasant experience. For example, staying at home can be an opportunity to watch movies that you have not had time to watch, play games, or read books that you like to read. Try to find something positive from this experience.

Have a routine while staying at home and make yourself live a life with structure, including getting up and going to bed at a normal hour, exercising and communicating with others regularly. Do something for your family, so that you can feel your self-worth. Stay in regular communication and do not avoid socializing.

However, if you are still feeling very low, not wanting to move, and have difficulty completing the most basic daily tasks, seek counseling from a professional psychiatrist.

Q: What should I do if I am anxious?

A: When staying at home, if you encounter an unexpected event, you will have anxiety and be overly worried and nervous about the future. When intervening, do not over-anticipate the future, and do not catastrophize an anticipated bad outcome. At all times, tell yourself "there is always a way", especially when you are very nervous or even show symptoms of somatization, such as panic, chest tightness, and sweating, do not panic, take deep breaths, play some soft piano music and focus your attention on something else; cook some simple food, do some simple chores, and avoid having all attention on yourself. If it is very urgent, you can go to the hospital for some basic tests to rule out physical illness and take some benzodiazepines under the guidance of a psychiatrist to alleviate anxiety.

Q: What should I do if I have insomnia?

A: Staying at home makes us prone to circadian rhythm disorders, and if you sleep too much during the day, you tend to have trouble sleeping at night. However, when depression and anxiety take over, it can also lead to insomnia, difficulty sleeping or waking up early.

Therefore, when you have difficulty sleeping, it is important to assess depression and anxiety, which may be part of the issue. A comprehensive assessment will facilitate a more comprehensive intervention and treatment in the early stage.

Insomnia is mainly induced by depression and anxiety, but sudden changes in the environment, excessive coffee or alcohol consumption can also induce difficulties falling asleep, waking up early or low sleep quality during the night, still feeling sleepy during the day, difficulty concentrating on studies or work, emotional instability, or reduced social functions.

When staying at home, if sleep problems persist, you can continuously record the time you go to bed, the time you fall asleep, the number of times you wake up during the night, the total number of hours you slept, the number of early wake-ups, and your mood and your ability to work during the day, which can be used to assist in assessing your mood and sleep conditions.

If you have sleep disorders, relax your mood, and do not exaggerate the problems caused by sleep. Try to avoid compensatory sleep during the day because of the difficulty sleeping at night. Instead, keep a regular lifestyle and follow your original routine.

Avoid overly intense exercises at night, listening to strong music or watching scary movies, spending too much time on your phone, and allow yourself to be in a quiet state to fall asleep. You can read a book before going to bed, and avoid lying in bed too early and waiting until time to sleep. Instead, get ready for bed when it's time to sleep. Do not anticipate the effects of sleep and be open to all sleep conditions. If the difficulty sleeping persists, you may get prescribed a small dose of sleep aid at the psychiatric department.

15、脂肪肝的小知识

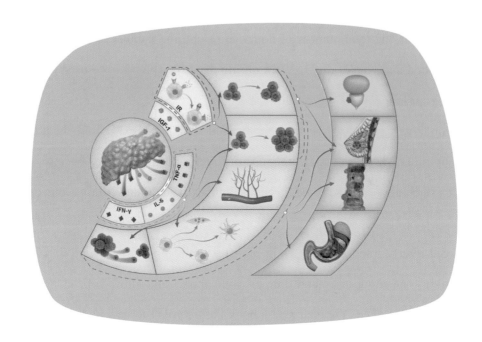

　　随着精细加工食品及各种甜品、饮料种类的增加，我们的味蕾也"欢乐"起来，下午茶已备受欢迎。此外，工作压力的增大及生活节奏的加快使得户外运动日益减少，超重、肥胖的人群逐渐增多。在出现这些外在表象时，真正的危害是同步伴随的内脏脂肪的堆积，其中较为常见的就是脂肪肝。

　　近年来，脂肪肝的患病率不断攀升，已成为全球第一大肝脏疾病。然而，无论是我国，还是发达国家的全科医生、非消化肝病专科医生，以及广大群众，至今仍对脂肪肝的危害，以及防治策略缺乏足够的认识。脂肪肝的预防和治疗的真正第一线，就在我们日常生活中。

Q： 何谓脂肪肝？

A： 通常我们所讲的脂肪肝，其完整的名称为非酒精性脂肪性肝病，最近被更名为代谢相关脂肪性肝病，是慢性肝病中较为常见的一种，其特征是肝细胞合成脂肪的能力增强，或转运脂肪入血的能力减退，肝细胞内大量脂滴堆积，即形成肝脂肪变。脂肪肝是各种原因引起的肝脏脂肪蓄积过多的一种病理状态。脂肪肝也有急性和慢性之分。前者通常起病急、病情重，表现为急性脂肪肝；后者起病隐匿，临床症状轻微且无特异性，表现为慢性脂肪肝。急性脂肪肝在临床上非常少见，目前日益增多的主要是慢性脂肪肝。

在慢性脂肪肝的发生和发展中，其主要由一种病因引起，也可以由多种病因同时作用或先后参与。肥胖、糖尿病是目前我国居民脂肪肝的主要病因，营养不良性脂肪肝仅流行于部分经济落后地区，遗传性疾病引起的代谢性脂肪肝非常少。

Q： 脂肪肝有哪些表现？

A： 脂肪肝是全身疾病累及肝脏的一种病理改变，其危害也不仅仅限于肝脏。脂肪肝是一种疾病，而不是亚健康。早期大部分患者无特异性的症状，有些人会出现肝区不适，少部分人会因为肝功能异常而出现食欲不佳、乏力等。脂肪肝常常合并肥胖、糖尿病、高脂血症、高血压、冠心病、痛风、胆结石、睡眠呼吸暂停综合征。

Q： 日常生活中常见的脂肪肝危险因素有哪些？

A： 不良生活方式是导致脂肪肝高发的最主要原因。要防治脂肪肝，必须从建立健康的生活方式做起，尤其是注意改善膳食结构。随着经济的发展，我国居民膳食结构和营养组成发生了明显变化，表现为粮食消耗量呈下降趋势，动物性食物消耗量成倍增长。人体热量和营养素的摄入量明显增加。高脂肪、高热量食品（包括含果糖饮料）消耗过多与肥胖症和脂肪肝关系密切。

特别是过量进食、喜甜食和荤食、常吃夜宵，以及不吃早餐等饮食习惯，为肥胖和脂肪肝的发病提供了条件。比起同等热量的早餐或午餐，一顿丰盛的晚餐更容易导致肥胖和脂肪肝。

另一个原因是多坐少动的生活方式。绝大多数脂肪肝患者习惯久坐，有些患者甚至从不参加体育运动。人体主要通过体力活动消耗多余热量，没有被消耗的热量会转化为脂肪储存。在肥胖的形成原因中，活动过少比摄食过多更重要。当脂肪沉积于皮下时，表现为肥胖；当脂肪堆积在肝脏时，就出现了脂肪肝。

Q: 如何预防脂肪肝的发生？

A: 脂肪肝的发生主要与肥胖、2 型糖尿病、酒精滥用等因素有关，故必须采取综合预防措施，才能收到较好效果。

首先，调整膳食结构，坚持以"植物性食物为主，动物性食物为辅，热量来源以粮食为主"的中国传统膳食方案，避免西方社会"高热量、高脂肪、高蛋白质、低纤维"膳食结构的缺陷，防止热量过剩，预防肥胖、糖尿病、高脂血症和脂肪肝的发生。在日常生活中，减少饮酒或戒酒。一日三餐定时、适量，早餐要吃饱，中餐要吃好，晚餐大半饱，避免吃得多、吃得快、吃零食、吃甜食、吃夜宵，以及把含糖饮料当水喝等不良习惯，以免热量摄入超标和扰乱机体代谢稳态，诱发肥胖、糖尿病和脂肪肝。

其次，"迈开腿"，进行中等量的有氧运动。人体对多余热量的利用，除转化为脂肪储存外，主要通过体力活动消耗。在肥胖，特别是内脏型肥胖的形成原因中，活动过少有时比摄食过多更为重要。根据自己的兴趣及时间分配选择适当的锻炼方式，建议无氧锻炼结合有氧锻炼，有氧锻炼可以进一步消耗多余的脂肪，降低体脂率，无氧锻炼可以增加骨骼肌的质量，防止肌少症，在一定程度上可以增高基础代谢率，也可使我们的身体更加健康。

Q: 脂肪肝与肿瘤是否相关？

A: 首当其冲的是肝癌。脂肪肝早期只是出现单纯的脂肪堆积；随着脂肪含量越来越高，可逐渐覆盖肝脏，使得肝脏容易发炎，进入脂肪性肝炎阶段；脂肪性肝炎反复发作，刺激肝脏中纤维组织增生，促使肝组织加厚变硬，进入肝硬化阶段；如果脂肪肝患者伴有高脂血症、肥胖和糖尿病等，则免疫功能受到损害，内环境紊乱，无法清除异常的细胞，久而久之发展成肝癌。

其次就是肝外肿瘤，有研究对 9.1 万人进行数据分析发现，脂肪肝患者结直肠癌患病风险增加。相关肿瘤还有前列腺癌、乳腺癌、胃癌等，需要人们在日常生活中积极防治和重视。

因此，平时应呵护好肝脏，保持心平气和、精神愉悦，若忍不住发脾气，不妨多喝菊花茶或绿茶等。每天保持充足的睡眠，应在 23 点之前入睡，使肝细胞得到足够的血液、营养和氧气滋养，促进肝细胞修复和再生。每天要有 30 分钟以上的运动，比如慢跑、打太极拳或八段锦等，把肝功能调整到最佳状态；补充足够的优质蛋白质以及维生素和微量元素，增强肝脏解毒和代谢能力。

15.Tips for fatty liver disease

Our taste buds have also changed with increased variety of fine processed foods, desserts and beverages. Afternoon tea has become very popular. Besides, the increased pressure at work and faster pace of life have led to a decrease in exercising outdoors, resulting in an increase in the number of people that are overweight or obese. This is only an external manifestation, as the real harm is the accumulation of visceral fat; a common condition is the fatty liver disease.

In recent years, the prevalence of patients with fatty liver disease has continued to increase; it has become the number one liver disease worldwide. However, general practitioners, herpetologists, and the general public in both China and developed countries still lack knowledge about the dangers of fatty liver disease and relevant prevention and treatment strategies. The real first line of defense and treatment of fatty liver disease is in our everyday life.

Q: *What is fatty liver disease?*

A: What we usually call fatty liver disease, which is non-alcoholic fatty liver disease in full, has recently been renamed metabolic-related fatty liver disease. It is one of the more common types of chronic liver diseases, characterized by an increase in the ability of liver cells to synthesize fat or a decrease in their ability to transport fat into the bloodstream, which results in the buildup of large amounts of lipid droplets in liver cells (i.e., hepatic steatosis). Fatty liver is a pathological condition due to excessive accumulation of fat in the liver from various causes. There is also a

distinction between acute and chronic fatty liver disease. The former usually has an acute onset, is severe and manifests as an acute fatty liver; the latter has an insidious onset, with mild and non-specific clinical symptoms, and manifests as a chronic fatty liver. Acute fatty liver disease is very rare clinically; nowadays, it is mainly chronic fatty liver disease that is increasing.

The development and progression of chronic fatty liver disease are mainly caused by one etiology but can also be caused by multiple etiologies simultaneously or sequentially. Obesity and diabetes are currently the major causes of fatty liver disease in the Chinese population; fatty liver disease due to malnutrition is only prevalent in some economically under-developed areas, and metabolic-associated fatty liver disease caused by hereditary diseases is very rare.

Q: *What are the signs of fatty liver disease?*

A: Fatty liver disease is a pathological change of systemic diseases involving the liver, and its damage is not only limited to the liver. Fatty liver disease is a disease, not suboptimal health. In the early stage, most patients have no specific symptoms, and some will experience discomfort in the liver area, poor appetite and fatigue due to abnormal liver function. It is often concomitant with obesity, diabetes, hyperlipidemia, hypertension, coronary heart disease, gout, gallstones, and sleep apnea syndrome.

Q: *What are the common risk factors for fatty liver disease in everyday life?*

A: An unhealthy lifestyle is the most important cause of the high incidence of fatty liver disease. To prevent and control fatty liver disease, it is necessary to start with establishing a healthy lifestyle, especially dietary structure. As the economy develops, dietary structure and nutritional composition of Chinese citizens have changed significantly, manifested by a decrease in grain consumption and an exponential increase in animal product consumption with significantly higher caloric and nutritional intake. Over–consumption of high–fat, high–calorie foods (including beverages containing fructose) is closely related to obesity and fatty liver disease.

In particular, overeating, preferring sweet and animal products, often eating late at night, and skipping breakfast all enable obesity and fatty liver disease to develop. A hearty dinner is more likely to lead to obesity and fatty liver disease than breakfast or lunch with the same amount of calories.

Sedentary lifestyle is the other cause. The vast majority of fatty liver disease patients are sedentary, and some never even participate in sports. The body burns excess calories mainly through physical activity, and the unburned calories are converted into fat to be stored. Among the causes of obesity, insufficient physical activity is more important than overeating. When fat is deposits under the skin, it manifests as obesity; when fat accumulates in the liver, it manifests as fatty liver disease.

Q: *How to prevent fatty liver disease?*

A: Fatty liver disease is mainly related to factors including obesity, type II diabetes and alcohol abuse. So, it is necessary to take comprehensive preventive measures to achieve better results.

Firstly, adjust the dietary structure, adhere to the traditional Chinese dietary plan of "plant–based food supplemented by animal products, with grain as the main source of calories", and avoid the defects of a western "high–calorie, high–fat, high–protein, and low–fiber" diet so as to avoid excess calories, and prevent obesity, diabetes, hyperlipidemia and fatty liver disease. In everyday life, reduce alcohol consumption or quit drinking, and have three meals a day at regular intervals and in moderation. Eat a full breakfast, a good lunch and a half–full dinner; avoid overeating, eating excessively fast, snacking, eating sweets, eating late at night, and consuming sugary drinks in place of water to avoid excessive caloric intake and disturbing the metabolic homeostasis, which can induce obesity, diabetes and fatty liver disease.

Secondly, do a moderate amount of aerobic exercises. Apart from converting the excess calories into fat to store, the body burns off excess calories mainly through physical activities. Among the causes of obesity, especially visceral obesity, insufficient physical activity is sometimes more important than overeating. Choose the appropriate exercise based on your own interests and time schedule. A combination of anaerobic and aerobic exercises is recommended, as aerobic exercises can further burn off excess fat and lower BMI, while anaerobic exercises can increase the mass of skeletal muscle, prevent sarcopenia, and increase the basal metabolic rate to some extent, thereby improving health.

Q: *Is fatty liver disease associated with tumors?*

A: First and foremost, liver cancer. In the early stage of fatty liver disease, there is only a simple buildup of fat; as the fat content increases, it can gradually cover the liver, making the liver rebel and inflame, which enters the stage of steatohepatitis; repeated onset of steatohepatitis stimulates the proliferation of fibrous tissue in the liver, prompting the liver tissue to thicken and harden, which enters the stage of cirrhosis. If patients with fatty liver disease also have other conditions such as hyperlipidemia, obesity and diabetes, their immune function is impaired, their bodies' internal environment is disordered, and abnormal cells cannot be removed, which leads to the development of liver cancer over time.

Secondly, extrahepatic tumors. A study analyzing data from 91000 individuals found that patients with fatty liver disease had an increased risk of colorectal cancer. There are also prostate, breast, and stomach cancer, which require active prevention and attention in everyday life.

Therefore, you should take care of your liver and stay calm and happy. If you can't help losing your temper, you should drink more chrysanthemum tea or green tea. Get enough sleep every day, in particular, fall asleep before 23:00. This allows liver cells to be nourished with enough blood, nutrients and oxygen to promote repair and regeneration. Exercise for more than 30 minutes every day, such as jogging, Tai Chi and Baduanjin, to adjust liver function to its optimal state. Consume sufficient high–quality protein as well as vitamins and trace elements to enhance the detoxification and metabolism of the liver.

16、药物性肝损伤不可忽视

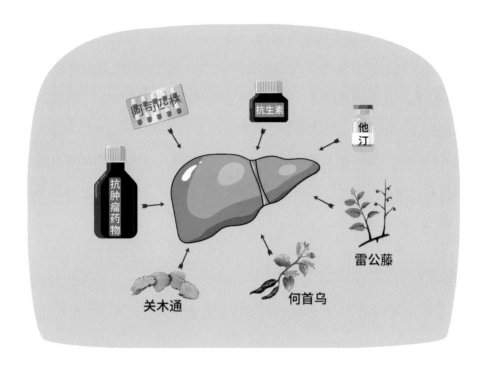

　　"药王"孙思邈的《备急千金要方》的自序中有一句话："凡欲治病，先以食疗，即食疗不愈，后乃药耳，是药三分毒。"当然，这里面所说的"毒"并非现在医学所指的"毒性"，而是指药物的偏性，但也说明了任何药物的使用都可能会导致与用药目的不相关的不良反应。

　　随着生活水平的提高，我们获得药物以及其他保健品的渠道更加多样、便捷，但同时也隐藏着许多问题。不少人认为小毛病不用上医院，而根据网上的建议自行购买、服用药物；或者听信广告宣传，通过网络购买保健品、营养品。殊不知，

"是药三分毒"，不少药物应用剂量过多时会引起肝脏不同程度的损伤。盲目用药不仅无益于治病，更可能损害健康。

Q: 什么是药物性肝损伤？

A: 肝脏是人体最大的解毒器官，临床所用药物绝大多数在肝脏进行代谢、转化、排泄。同时，身体内各种代谢的终末产物及毒物等也通过肝脏来进行解毒处理。因此，在不规范服药，或不注意监测肝功能情况的时候，肝脏很容易受到药物的损害。临床上，药物性肝损伤的发生率为 1.4% ～ 8.1%，占急性肝损伤住院患者的 20%，是临床上常见的药物不良反应之一，从总体数据看占比不高，但却很重要。如果不能早期及时发现和治疗，不定期监测，放任肝功能不全持续进展，甚至可能危及生命。

Q: 哪些药物会导致肝损伤？

A: 已知全球有 1100 多种上市药物具有潜在的肝毒性，常见的包括如下几种。

（1）非甾体抗炎药，如阿司匹林、对乙酰氨基酚、双氯芬酸等。

（2）心血管药物，如他汀类（阿托伐他汀、辛伐他汀）。

（3）精神类药物，如氯丙嗪、奥氮平等。

（4）抗菌药物，如抗结核类（利福平、异烟肼）、抗真菌药物（氟康唑、伏立康唑）、大环内酯类（红霉素、克拉霉素）、氯霉素、四环素等。

（5）抗肿瘤药物，如环磷酰胺、甲氨蝶呤、阿霉素、依托泊苷等。

（6）中草药类，如关木通、雷公藤、何首乌等。

除了这些常见药，生活中还有很大一部分肝损伤来自老年人喜爱的保健品、健身爱好者的蛋白粉、美容达人的美白丸，甚至还有贴在皮肤上的药膏、粉刷新家的油漆等，都在悄悄影响着我们的健康。

Q： 药物性肝损伤有哪些表现？

A： 药物引起的急性肝炎通常会发生在用药后的 1～4 周，症状与其他肝炎大致相同，常见表现如下。

（1）疲乏、食欲不振。

（2）恶心呕吐、厌食。

（3）发热、恶寒。

（4）皮肤、巩膜、小便黄染。

（5）肝区不适。

进一步就诊可见肝肿大伴有压痛、转氨酶升高、血常规中嗜酸性粒细胞水平升高；严重时出现黄疸、凝血机制障碍、肝性脑病、上消化道出血，有可能危及生命。因此，一旦出现以上症状，应积极就医治疗。

Q： 日常生活中，如何早期识别药物性肝损伤？

A： 如果没有基础肝病，有可疑肝损伤药物的服用史，伴随出现肝损伤的临床表现，需要高度警惕是否已出现药物性肝损伤。除了有上述症状出现外，部分患者在早期没有任何不适的症状，但肝功能的异常在悄然发生着。因此，倘若在某些疾病的治疗过程中，需要服用影响肝功能的药物，如化疗患者，则需要定期监测肝功能，做到早发现、早诊断、早治疗。

Q： 怀疑出现药物性肝损伤后，是否即刻停用可疑药物？

A： 药物性肝损伤为排他性诊断，需要根据肝损伤的程度及所服用药物的必要性，权衡利弊后再决定是否停用。虽然临床上急性药物性肝损伤占绝大多数，但仍有6%～20%可发展成慢性，故需引起重视。在治疗原发性疾病的同时，兼顾肝功能的状态。

16.Drug-induced liver injury should not be ignored

In the preface of the *Valuable Prescriptions for Emergency* by Sun Simiao, the "King of Medicine", there is a sentence that says, "Whenever you want to cure a disease, first treat it with food remedies. If the condition has not improved, then use medication. Every medication has its poison." Of course, the "poison" mentioned here is not the "toxicity" referred to in modern medicine, but it refers to the property of the drugs, but it also points out that any medication have side effects that is not related to are purpose or function.

As the standard of living improves, there is more diverse and convenient access to medicine and other health products, but at the same time, there are many hidden issues. Many people think that they don't need to go to the hospital for minor issues and can purchase and take medication on their own according to online advice; or they trust the advertisements and buy health and nutrition products on the Internet. However, they are not aware that "every drug has its side effects" and that different doses and types of drugs can cause different degrees of liver injury. Using medication arbitrarily is not only unhelpful but may also damage your health.

Q: *What is the drug-induced liver injury?*

A: The liver is the largest detoxification organ in the human body, and the majority of drugs in clinical practice are metabolized, transformed and excreted in the liver. At the same time, various end products of metabolism and toxins in the body are also detoxified and processed through the liver. Therefore, when medications are not taken correctly or liver function is not monitored, the liver is prone to drug-induced injuries. Clinically, the incidence of drug-reduced liver injury is 1.4%-8.1%, accounting for 20% of hospitalized patients with acute liver injury, and it is one of the common adverse drug reactions in clinical practice. Although the proportion is not high, it is very important. If it is not detected or treated early and in the early stage in a timely manner or goes without regular monitoring, hepatic insufficiency can progress to become life-threatening.

Q: What drugs can cause a loss of liver function?

A: More than 1100 marketed drugs worldwide are known to have potential hepatotoxicity. The common ones are as follows.

(1) Nonsteroidal anti-inflammatory drugs, such as aspirin, acetaminophen and diclofenac.

(2) Cardiovascular drugs, such as statins (atorvastatin and simvastatin).

(3) Psychotropic drugs, such as chlorpromazine and olanzapine.

(4) Antibacterial drugs, such as anti-tuberculosis drugs (rifampin and isoniazid), antifungal drugs (fluconazole and voriconazole), macrolides (erythromycin and clarithromycin), chloramphenicol and tetracycline.

(5) Anti-tumor drugs, such as cyclophosphamide, methotrexate, adriamycin and etoposide.

(6) Traditional Chinese herbs, such as manshurian dutchmanspipe stem, thunder god vine and fleeceflower root.

In addition to these common drugs, a large percentage of liver injury in everyday life is due to health products favored by the elderly, protein powder for fitness enthusiasts, whitening pills for beauty experts, and even ointments for external use, and paints used in a new home, all of which are quietly affecting our health.

Q: *What are the signs of drug-related liver injury?*

A: Drug-induced acute hepatitis usually occurs 1-4 weeks after drug administration, and the symptoms are roughly the same as other hepatitis, with common symptoms as follows.

(1) Fatigue, loss of appetite.

(2) Nausea and vomiting, anorexia.

(3) Fever and chills.

(4) Jaundice and yellowing urine.

(5) Discomfort in the liver area.

Further consultation may reveal enlarged liver with pressure pain, elevated transaminases, and elevated eosinophils in the blood; in severe cases, high jaundice, coagulation disorder, hepatic encephalopathy, and upper gastrointestinal bleeding may occur, which can be life-threatening. Therefore, if any of the above symptoms appear, you should seek medical treatment.

Q: *How can I recognize drug-induced liver injury early in everyday life?*

A: If there is a history of suspected liver-damaging drugs without underlying liver disease, concomitant with clinical manifestations of impaired liver function, you should be on high alert that drug-induced liver injury may have developed. Other than the symptoms mentioned above, some patients do not have any discomfort in the early stage, but hepatic insufficiency is quietly present. Therefore, if you need to take medication that affects liver function during the treatment of certain diseases, such as chemotherapy, monitor your liver function closely and regularly to achieve early detection, diagnosis and treatment.

Q: *Should the suspicious drug be stopped immediately if drug-induced liver injury is suspected?*

A: Drug-induced liver injury is an exclusive diagnosis, and the extent of liver damage needs to be weighed against the necessity of the drug to make a decision. Also, the most important is the consultation and evaluation with the primary care physician. Although acute drug-induced liver injury accounts for the majority of clinical cases, there are still 6%–20% that can develop into a chronic injury, so it needs to be taken seriously. Take into account liver condition while treating the primary disease.

17、脑卒中的小知识

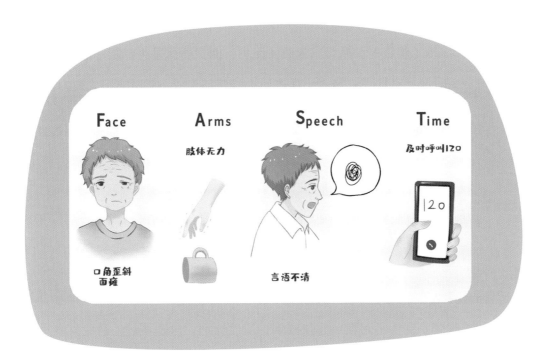

Q： 什么是脑卒中？

A： 脑卒中（cerebral stroke）又称脑血管意外、中风，是一种急性脑血管疾病，是由于脑部血管突然破裂或因血管阻塞导致血液不能流入大脑组织而引起脑组织损伤的一组疾病，分别被称为出血性脑卒中（脑出血）和缺血性脑卒中（脑梗死）。其中，脑梗死占脑卒中总数的 60% ~ 70%，而脑出血的死亡率更高。

Q: 出现哪些症状需要警惕脑卒中？

A: 牢记"FAST"规则，一旦怀疑发生脑卒中，迅速就医很重要。

F——Face（脸）：是否出现一侧口角歪斜，面部下坠？做微笑表情时两边是否对称？

A——Arms（胳膊）：是否出现肢体无力？两只胳膊是否都能一样抬举？

S——Speech（言语）：是否出现讲话不清楚，或者不能听懂别人说的话？

T——Time（时间）：如果你出现了上述任何一种症状，抓紧时间，赶紧拨打"120"或到最近的医院急诊科就诊。

Q: 我还没发生过脑卒中，我需要如何预防脑卒中的发生？

A: 需要做到以下四点。

（1）合理饮食，控制体重：多吃粗粮及五谷；适当多吃新鲜的瓜果蔬菜；吃适量的奶制品、肉、鱼、蛋及豆类；少吃油、糖、盐类。

（2）改变不良生活习惯：建议戒烟，适度饮酒；早睡早起，避免熬夜；加强身体锻炼，居家生活期间选择适合自己的锻炼方式，如瑜伽、打太极拳、做有氧运动等。

（3）了解自己的血压、血糖、血脂，控制危险因素。

控制血压：血压应维持在低于 140/90 mmHg，有糖尿病及高脂血症的患者血压应低于 130/80 mmHg。应规律服用适当的降压药物，监测血压。

控制血糖：空腹血糖浓度应低于 8.8 mmol/L，餐后 2 小时血糖浓度应低于 11.1 mmol/L；监测血糖，规律科学地服用降糖药物。

控制血脂：甘油三酯及胆固醇降至正常范围，中老年人低密度脂蛋白胆固醇（LDL-C）小于 3.1 mmol/L，规律服用调脂药物。

（4）其他高危因素的控制：若有心房颤动、心脏瓣膜病、高凝状态等基础疾病，居家生活期间仍需要按照预防脑卒中的方案规律服药。

Q：若已经是脑卒中患者，居家生活期间该怎么做？

A：首先，区分是出血性脑卒中还是缺血性脑卒中，这很重要。

出血性脑卒中：保持情绪稳定，监测血压，积极控制血压，规律服药，不随意增减药量；适量活动，加强对患肢或语言功能的康复训练；合理调配饮食。

缺血性脑卒中：监测血压、血糖，规律服药，不随意增减药量；规律服用抗凝药物（或抗血小板药物）+ 他汀类药物预防脑卒中的再发；适量活动，加强对患肢或语言功能的康复训练；合理调配饮食。

Q：若发生了脑卒中，有哪些治疗方法？

A：若出现脑卒中症状，及时拨打"120"就诊。完善头颅 CT 检查及血液检查，鉴别出血性或缺血性脑卒中。

若为出血性脑卒中：

（1）手术治疗：根据出血部位及出血量评估是否有手术指征；基底节中等量出血（壳核出血 ≥ 30 mL，丘脑出血 ≥ 15 mL），小脑出血（出血量 ≥ 10 mL，或直径 ≥ 3 cm），需积极考虑手术治疗，及时清除血肿。大量出血或形成脑疝者，需急诊行去骨瓣减压血肿清除术，以挽救生命。

（2）内科治疗：对于无手术指征的患者，均需要积极进行内科治疗。监测血压，早期降压治疗，收缩期血压降至 140 mmHg 以下是安全的。止血药物疗效不确定，不推荐。积极对因治疗及防治并发症。

若为缺血性脑卒中：

（1）静脉溶栓治疗：对于发病时间在 4.5 小时以内，无溶栓禁忌的患者，推荐使用阿替普酶（0.9 mg/kg）静脉溶栓治疗。超过 4.5 小时者，需行影像学检查评估缺血半暗带大小以决定静脉溶栓是否获益。

（2）急诊血管内取栓治疗：对于发病时间短于 6 小时的患者，行头颅 CTA 检查即头部血管成像检查或 MRA 检查明确血管情况，评估取栓指征；对于发病 6 ～ 16 小时的患者，完善多模态 CTA 检查筛选是否有取栓指征。

（3）对于无静脉溶栓或血管内取栓治疗指征的患者，根据患者临床症状的轻重及病因选择抗血小板 + 他汀或抗凝 + 他汀二级预防。

（4）早期康复治疗。

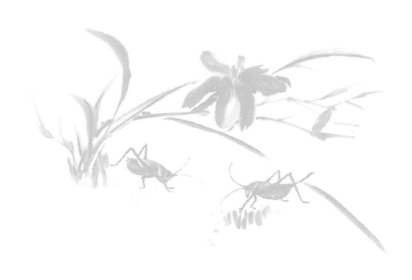

17.Tips for cerebral stroke

Q: What is the cerebral stroke?

A: Cerebral stroke is also known as cerebrovascular accident and stroke. It is an acute cerebrovascular disease, which is a group of diseases caused by the sudden rupture of blood vessels in the brain or the blockage of blood vessels, resulting in the inability of blood to flow into the brain tissues, causing brain tissue damage. These are called hemorrhagic stroke and ischemic stroke, respectively. Among these, ischemic stroke accounts for 60% − 70% of all strokes, while the hemorrhagic stroke has a higher mortality rate.

Q: What symptoms are alerts for a stroke?

A: It is important to remember the "FAST" rule and to seek medical attention as soon as a stroke is suspected.

F—Face: Does one side of the mouth appear crooked, and is the face dropping? Is the grin symmetrical?

A—Arms: Is there limb weakness? Can both arms be lifted equally?

S—Speech: Is there unclear speech, or an inability to understand what others are saying?

T—Time: If you experience any of the above symptoms, call "120" or go to the emergency department of the nearest hospital as soon as possible.

Q: I haven't had a stroke yet; what do I need to do to prevent one?

A: Pay attention to the following points.

(1) Eat a balanced diet and control your weight: Eat more coarse grains and fresh fruits and vegetables; consume moderate amounts of dairy products, meat, fish, eggs and beans; consume less oil, sugar and salt.

(2) Try to get rid of bad habits: It is recommended to quit smoking, drink moderately, go to bed early and wake up early, avoid staying up late, exercise more and choose suitable types of exercises for yourself when staying at home, such as yoga, Tai Chi and aerobic exercises.

(3) Know your blood pressure, blood sugar, blood lipids and control risk factors.

Blood pressure control: Blood pressure should be maintained below 140/90 mmHg, and below 130/80 mmHg for patients with diabetes and hyperlipidemia. You should take appropriate antihypertensive medication and regularly monitor blood pressure.

Blood sugar control: Normal blood levels should be lower than 8.8 mmol/L when fasting and lower than 11.1 mmol/L 2 hours after eating. You should monitor your blood sugar level and take hypoglycemic medication appropriately.

Cholesterol control: The target is to lower triglycerides and cholesterol to normal range, and low-density lipoprotein cholesterol (LDL-C) to less than 3.1 mmol/L. You should take cholesterol-regulating medication regularly.

(4) Control of other risk factors: If you have underlying conditions such as atrial fibrillation, valvular heart disease, and hypercoagulable state, you should continue to

take your medication regularly following the stroke prevention protocol when staying at home.

Q: *If I have already had a stroke, what should I do when staying at home?*

A: First, it is important to distinguish hemorrhagic stroke and ischemic stroke.

Hemorrhagic stroke: Maintain emotional stability, monitor and actively control blood pressure; take medication regularly, and do not increase or decrease the dosage arbitrarily. Moderately exercise and continue the rehabilitation of the affected limb or improve speech function. A healthy diet is also important for recovery.

Ischemic stroke: Monitor blood pressure and blood sugar levels; take medication regularly and do not increase or decrease the dosage arbitrarily; take anticoagulant drugs (or antiplatelet drugs) + statin drugs regularly to prevent the recurrence of stroke. Moderately exercise and continue the rehabilitation of the affected limbs or speech function. Eat a healthy diet.

Q: *If a stroke occurs, what are the treatments available?*

A: Call "120" for emergency medical care if you develop stroke symptoms. Complete head CT scan and blood tests to identify whether the stroke is hemorrhagic or ischemic.

If it is hemorrhagic stroke.

(1) Surgery: The indication for surgery will be assessed based on the site and amount of bleeding. Moderate bleeding in the basal ganglia($\geqslant$ 30 mL in the

putamen and $\geqslant 15$ mL in the thalamus) and cerebellar bleeding (volume $\geqslant 10$ mL, or diameter $\geqslant 3$ cm) require surgery for the timely removal of the hematoma. In cases of massive bleeding or brain herniation formation, emergency bone flap decompression and hematoma removal are required to save lives.

(2) Internal medicine treatment: Treatment at internal medicine is needed for all patients without surgical indications. Monitor blood pressure and use early−stage antihypertensive therapy to lower it to below 140 mmHg, which is the safe range. The efficacy of hemostatic drugs is uncertain. So they are not recommended. Conduct etiological treatment and prevention of complications.

If it is ischemic stroke.

(1) Intravenous thrombolytic therapy: For patients with an onset time of less than 4.5 hours and no contraindication to thrombolysis, intravenous thrombolytic therapy with alteplase (0.9 mg/kg) is recommended. For an onset time longer than 4.5 hours, imaging is required to assess the size of the ischemic penumbra to determine whether intravenous thrombolytic therapy will be beneficial.

(2) Emergency endovascular embolization: For patients with an onset of less than 6 hours, cranial CTA or MRA will be performed to clarify the vascular condition and assess the indicators for embolization; for patients with an onset of 6−16 hours, multimodal CTA will be completed to screen indicators for embolization.

(3) For patients without intravenous thrombolysis or endovascular thrombolysis indications, antiplatelet + statin or anticoagulation + statin secondary prevention will be chosen based on the severity of the patient's clinical symptoms and causes.

(4) Early rehabilitation.

18、手抖与帕金森病的关系

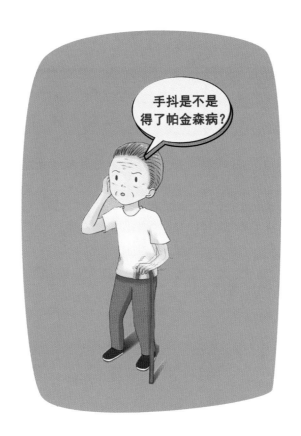

Q： 什么是手抖？

A： 手抖又被称为手部震颤，是一种非自主的、有节律的肌肉收缩而产生的手部抖动。除了最常见的手部，其他部位包括手臂、头部、声带、躯干和腿均可以发生震颤。可以单独出现，也可以多个部位一起出现，任何年龄都可以发生，但在中老年人中最为常见；可以是间断性的，也可以是持续性的。

Q: 突然出现手科，应该怎么排查原因？

A: 有以下两大类原因。

(1) 一般已知的原因：

①某些药物的影响，如哮喘药物、苯丙胺、皮质类固醇和其他治疗精神和神经疾病的药物。

②摄入酒精或含咖啡因的饮料。

③药物戒断：如镇静催眠类药物。

④缺乏睡眠。

⑤压力大、焦虑、情绪过激。

(2) 疾病相关的原因：

①甲状腺功能亢进。

②肝、肾功能衰竭。

③焦虑或恐慌。

④脑卒中。

⑤神经变性疾病，如帕金森病或特发性震颤。

Q: 出现手科，我应该怎么自我保健？

A: 可以尝试以下三种方法。

(1) 避免压力和练习放松技巧。

(2) 保证充足的睡眠。

(3) 避免过量饮酒和摄入咖啡因。

Q: 出现手抖，什么情况需要咨询医生或就诊？

A: 出现以下情况需要求助医生，优先就诊科室为神经内科：第一次出现手抖，且经过自我保健仍不能缓解；长时间无法控制的手抖；同时有平衡问题或感觉丧失。

Q: 帕金森病的手抖加重了该怎么办？

A: 手抖是帕金森病的常见症状，居家生活期间，应该规律服药，不中断药物。若规律服药，手抖或帕金森病症状仍然加重，需要按照以下流程操作。

(1) 观察是否有加重手抖症状的病因：如感冒、发热等生病状态，睡眠不充分，焦虑或抑郁情绪，低血糖等。

(2) 若无明显的诱因，或者经过一般的保健处理，手抖症状仍无好转，需要考虑帕金森病进展或疗效减退，应咨询专科医生调整药物方案。

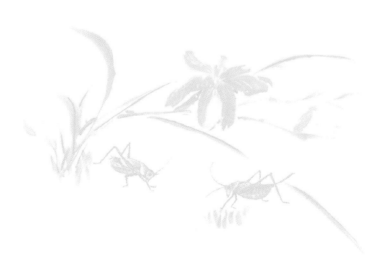

18. The relationship between shaking hands and Parkinson's disease

Q: What is shaking hands?

A: Shaking hands, also known as tremor, is an involuntary, rhythmic muscle contraction that produces shaking movement in the hands. In addition to the hands, which are the most common, tremors can occur in other areas, including the arms, head, vocal cords, trunk and legs. They can occur alone or in multiple sites together, on people of any age, but is most common in the middle-aged and elderly. It can be intermittent or constant.

Q: What should I do to find out the cause of sudden shaking hands?

A: There are two main categories of causes for this.

(1) Common, known causes.

① The effects of certain medications, such as asthma medications, amphetamines, corticosteroids and other medications used to treat psychiatric and neurological disorders.

② Alcohol consumption or caffeine intake.

③ Drug withdrawal, e.g., sedative-hypnotics.

④ Lack of sleep.

⑤ Stress, anxiety, and emotional overstimulation.

(2) Disease−related causes.

① Hyperthyroidism.

② Liver and kidney failure.

③ Anxiety or panic.

④ Stroke.

⑤ Neurodegenerative diseases, such as Parkinson's disease and essential tremor.

Q: *What should I do for self−care when I have shaking hands?*

A: You can try the following three approaches.

(1) Avoid stress and practice relaxation techniques.

(2) Ensure adequate sleep.

(3) Avoid excessive alcohol consumption and caffeine intake.

Q: *What conditions require medical consultation when I have shaking hands?*

A: The following conditions require immediate medical attention, neurology department first: Shaking hands occur for the first time and are not relieved by self−care; uncontrollable shaking hands for a long period of time; tremors concomitant with balance issues or loss of sensation.

Q: *What should I do if the shaking hands due to Parkinson's disease has worsened?*

A: Shaking hands is a common symptom of Parkinson's disease.When staying at home, you also should take medications regularly without interruption. If you take your medication regularly and your shaking hands or Parkinson's symptoms has still worsened, you need to follow the procedures below.

(1) See if there are causes that aggravate the tremors: illness such as flu and fever, inadequate sleep, anxiety or depression, and low blood sugar.

(2) If there is no clear trigger, or if shaking hands do not get better after general healthcare treatment, consider the progression of Parkinson's disease or the diminishing efficacy of the treatment, and consult a specialist to adjust the medication regimen.

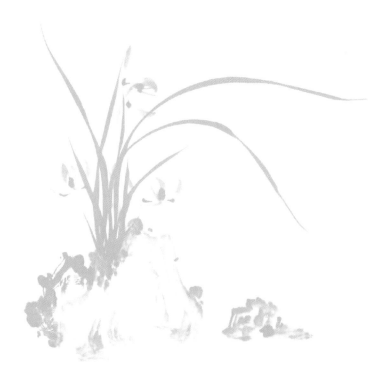

19、发现泡沫尿该怎么办

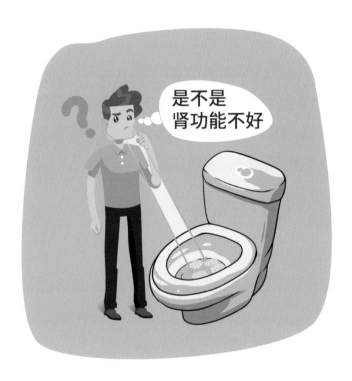

Q: 什么是泡沫尿？

A: 泡沫尿就是指尿液中出现很多气泡。尿液中泡沫的形成是由于尿液表面张力高所致，张力越高，形成的泡沫越多，而表面张力的大小又跟尿液的成分有关。人体的血液流经肾脏的肾小球时经过滤形成原尿，再流经肾小管时，原尿中对人体有用的全部葡萄糖、大部分水分和无机盐被肾小管重吸收回到肾小管周围毛细血管的血液中，剩余的水、无机盐、尿素、尿酸等物质就形成了尿液。因此正常人体尿液中所含物质较少，其表面张力不大，不足以形成众多泡沫。如果尿液中的一些成分，如有机物质和无机物质相对增多，那么尿液的表面张力就会相应增高，此时尿液的泡沫就会增多。

Q： 出现泡沫尿一定是生病了吗？

A： 不一定。很多生理性情况也会出现尿液泡沫增多。

（1）尿液浓缩：尤其是晨尿、剧烈运动以及腹泻、出汗等情况导致机体缺水时，可使尿液浓缩，尿液原有成分比例相对增高。

（2）大量饮酒或食用过多的高蛋白食物，或服用某些药物，导致尿液成分改变。

（3）男性精液、前列腺液、尿道黏液，女性白带、经血等混入尿液，使尿液中成分增多而形成泡沫尿。

（4）尿急或排尿压力加大，尿速增快，也可见泡沫增多，但这类泡沫一般在静置后可很快消散。

（5）便池或接尿容器中混入一些洗涤剂等。

以上这些情况形成的泡沫尿并非疾病导致，去除相关因素后可恢复正常。

Q： 哪些疾病会导致泡沫尿发生？

A： 以下情况属于病理性泡沫尿。

（1）蛋白尿：正常人尿液中是没有蛋白质的，当尿液中出现大量的蛋白质时，就会在尿液表面形成细密、量多、经久不散的泡沫，这种泡沫尿一般称为"蛋白尿"。蛋白尿是各种肾病患者常见的症状之一，包括各种肾炎、肾病综合征等。严重的肾脏疾病，除存在蛋白尿外，还可能有尿素排出增多、尿比重增加或出现管型尿等。

（2）泌尿系统疾病：泌尿系感染、结石、肿瘤或一些特殊疾病（如膀胱结肠瘘等），可以使尿道中炎性分泌物增多或尿液成分发生改变，尿中泡沫增多，若感染的是一些产气细菌，会让尿液产生大量气泡。

（3）尿糖增多：糖尿病患者若血糖控制欠佳，尿糖或尿酮体含量升高，可导致尿中泡沫增多。短时间内静脉输入大量葡萄糖，超过肾糖阈而出现一过性尿糖增多，也会导致泡沫尿。另有一部分糖尿病患者服用通过尿中排糖来降低血糖浓度的新型降糖药物，导致尿糖增多（这种情况需与糖尿病肾病的蛋白尿相鉴别）。

（4）尿液酸碱度改变：高尿酸血症或痛风患者，尿酸排出增多导致尿液酸碱度发生改变，也会出现泡沫尿。

（5）肝脏疾病：部分肝脏疾病如阻塞性黄疸和肝细胞性黄疸，尿胆红素水平升高，尿液呈豆油样改变，振荡后出现黄色泡沫且不易消失。

Q: 出现泡沫尿，我们应该怎么办？

A: 出现泡沫尿后我们不能忽视，也不用过度惊慌而随意求医或盲目吃药，关键是要找到原因。经改善饮食、饮水习惯等生活方式后，如仍存在泡沫尿，需要到医院进一步检查，可以检查的项目有尿常规（初筛）、尿微量白蛋白/尿肌酐比值（确诊）、24小时尿蛋白定量（定量检测）。如果出现泡沫尿，并且伴有水肿、肉眼血尿、夜尿增多、血压高、糖尿病等情况，一定要及时到肾内科就诊，不要耽误了治疗时机。

19.What should I do if I find foamy urine

Q: What is foamy urine?

A: Foamy urine refers to when there are many bubbles in the urine. The formation of foam in urine is due to the high surface tension of urine; the higher the tension, the more foam there will be, and the level of surface tension, in turn, is related to the content of urine. Urine in a human body is formed through the following process. Blood flows through the glomerulus of the kidney and after filtration forms primary urine. Then, it flows through the renal tubules where all the glucose, most of the water and inorganic salts in the primary urine that are useful to the body are reabsorbed by the renal tubules back into the blood in the capillaries around the renal tubules. The remaining water, inorganic salts, urea, uric acid and other substances make up urine. Therefore, normal human urine contains little material, and its surface tension is not high enough to form a lot of foam. If there is a relative increase in some content in urine, such as organic and inorganic substances, the surface tension of urine will increase correspondingly, and the amount of foam will also increase in urine.

Q: Does the presence of foamy urine mean that I am sick?

A: Not necessarily. Many other physiological conditions can also lead to an increase of foam in urine.

(1) Higher concentration of urine: Especially morning urine, strenuous exercise,

and dehydration, such as diarrhea and sweating, can lead to the higher concentration of urine and a relative increase in the proportion of the original content in the urine.

(2) Drinking large amounts of alcohol, consuming too much high–protein food, or taking certain medications can change the content in the urine.

(3) When semen, prostate fluid, and urethral mucus of male, or leukorrhea and menstruation of female are mixed into the urine, it will increase the content in the urine and lead to foamy urine.

(4) Urinary urgency or increased pressure to urinate, and increased speed of urination can also lead to visible bubbles in the urine, but these bubbles generally dissipate quickly after the urine has settled.

(5) There may also be detergent or other substances in the urinal or urine containers.

The increase of foam in urine in these cases is not caused by a disease and it can return to normal after taking out relevant factors.

Q: What diseases can cause foamy urine?

A: The following are considered pathological foamy urine.

(1) Proteinuria: There is no protein in normal urine, but when there is high protein content in the urine, it will form large amounts of fine foam on the urine surface, which will not dissipate for a long time. Proteinuria is one of the common symptoms in patients with kidney diseases, including nephritis and nephrotic syndrome. Severe kidney diseases can also lead to increased urea excretion, increased urine specific gravity or the appearance of urinary casts in addition to proteinuria.

(2) Urologic diseases: Urinary tract infections, stones, tumors or some other diseases (such as colovesical fistula) can increase inflammation in the urethra or change urine content, making the urine foamy, especially if the infection is due to clostridia, which can lead to large amounts of bubbles in the urine.

(3) Increased glucose in urine: For diabetic patients with poor glycemic control, the increase of glucose and ketone in urine can lead to more foam. This can also be seen as a result of consuming large amounts of carbohydrates in a short period of time or intravenous infusion of large amounts of glucose that exceeds the renal glucose threshold, resulting in a transient increase in glucose in urine and thus foamy urine. Other diabetic patients who take the newer glucose-lowering drugs that lower blood glucose by excreting sugar through the urine can experience increased glucose in urine (This condition needs to be distinguished from proteinuria in diabetic nephropathy).

(4) Altered urine pH: In patients with hyperuricemia or gout, increased uric acid excretion leads to altered urine pH, which can also lead to foamy urine.

(5) Liver diseases: Some liver diseases, such as obstructive jaundice and hepatocellular jaundice can lead to elevated urinary bilirubin and an oil-like change of texture in urine; yellow foam will appear in the urine after shaking and does not disappear easily.

Q: What should we do if we have foamy urine?

A: When foamy urine appears, we should not ignore it, or be overly alarmed to seek medical help arbitrarily or take medication blindly. The key is to find the cause. If foamy urine is still present after lifestyle changes, such as improved eating and drinking habits, you need to go to the hospital for further examination, such as urine routine (primary screening), urine microalbumin/urine albumin−creatinine ratio (confirming the diagnosis), and 24−hour urine protein test (quantification). If foamy urine occurs with swelling, visible hematuria, increased nocturia, high blood pressure and diabetes, it is important to seek timely medical help at the nephrology department without delaying treatment.

20、高血压相关知识

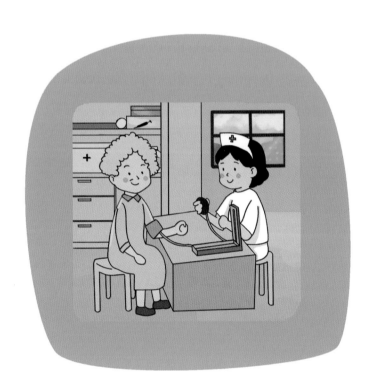

Q: 居家生活期间如何正确监测血压？

A: 坚持规律地监测血压很关键，有利于及时发现血压波动，并且将数据提供给医生作为调整用药的依据。最新的国际指南推荐用电子血压计测量血压，监测血压时应在休息30分钟后平静状态下测量，测量3次取平均值。一般以肱动脉处测的血压为主要参考，因此需要选用臂式血压计，使用的时候认真阅读说明书，根据设备说明使用袖带，在刚开始进行高血压治疗时，或者刚调整过药物剂量者，应每日起床后（饭前）、睡觉前各测 1 次，直到至少连续 1 周血压都能稳定达标后，再减少频率。血压控制得很好的患者，每周测 1 ～ 2 次，选在自己每日血压较高的时候进行测量，通常是晨起时。

Q： 高血压患者居家生活期间如何注意饮食偏嗜？

A： 避免饮食不节：避免饮食肥腻、甜腻、过咸，每人每日食盐摄入量不超过 6 g（一啤酒瓶盖），注意隐性盐的摄入（咸菜、鸡精、酱油等）。戒烟戒酒：烟可损伤脉管，导致气虚血瘀，诱发经络不畅、不通；酒可影响脾气运化，引起痰浊内生，均可引起血压的波动、眩晕症状的发生与加重。《本草纲目》曰："春食凉，夏食寒，以养阳；秋食温，冬食热，以养阴。"春夏阳盛，故宜食寒凉抑制亢阳避免伤阴；秋冬阴盛，宜食温热抑制盛阴而保全阳气。在立秋之后，饮食应该开始慢慢过渡，为迎接秋冬的寒冷打好基础。夏季主"长"，秋季主"收"，立秋之后，环境逐渐从湿润转为干燥，饮食应避免过燥过热、辛散之品，如姜、辣椒、花椒、桂皮，过食易伤阴，适当服用平和凉润、酸甘之品，如蜂蜜、百合、葡萄、柚子等。

Q： 高血压患者居家生活期间如何进行体育锻炼、控制体重？

A： 体育锻炼、增强体质：规律的中等强度运动（如快走、打太极拳、八段锦等常见健身方式）均有直接的降压效果，可改善眩晕症状，可以每次 30 分钟，每周 5 ～ 7 次，可使收缩压下降 4 ～ 9 mmHg。肥胖者居家也要继续减轻体重：肥胖者多痰湿，常伴随脾虚，脾胃运化无力，酿湿生痰，痰浊阻滞气血运行可引发清气上升，出现头晕等症状。每减重 10 kg 可使收缩压下降 5 ～ 20 mmHg。一般要求 BMI<24 kg/m²，腰围 <90 cm（男）或 <85

cm(女)。避免久坐久卧。

Q: 高血压患者居家生活期间为什么要保持情绪稳定、劳逸结合？

A: 居家生活期间，高血压患者尤其要注意保持情绪稳定、防止七情内伤：喜怒忧思恐等均可伤及脏腑，比如大怒引起肝风煽动，情志抑郁日久耗伤心肾，导致阴气不足，进而引起目昏耳鸣、震眩不定，可表现为血压波动明显，甚至血压过高引起脑卒中。因此保持心情愉快、心境柔和，可避免血压的波动，控制病情进展。过劳会影响神经系统对血压的调节，熬夜可能使交感、副交感系统调节功能紊乱，导致血压波动；中医认为过劳伤阴血、伤气，阴血亏虚会并发阳亢，气虚会引起痰浊、痰饮，发生眩晕；因此倡导脑力劳动与体力劳动结合，避免过劳、熬夜。

Q: 夏秋之交，血压波动，居家生活期间如何调整睡眠时间？

A: 到了秋天就应该开始收敛体内阳气，相较于春、夏两季适当延长睡眠时间，通过充足的睡眠收敛自身的精气，以缓和秋天的肃杀之气。充足的睡眠有利于内分泌、激素的调节，帮助血压平稳。高血压患者如在查找到原因和经调节情志后仍不能很好地睡眠，建议适当使用助眠药物或者中医治疗调理。建议每日晚上 10 点前入睡，保证每日睡眠时间不少于 7 小时，但不宜超过 9 小时。

Q: 居家生活期间如何正确使用中药代茶饮？

A: 高血压患者如能至医院门诊就诊，可由中医问诊后辨证施治，开具中药处方调节阴阳平衡，补虚泄实，从而起到降低血压、改善症状的作用。

如不能定时至门诊就诊或无法坚持口服汤药，可酌情选择一些常见药物适量代茶饮用，或磨粉每日适量温水兑服，具体用量可通过互联网医院咨询专业医生。

代茶药物的选择要点如下：肝阳上亢者如面红、头目胀痛、易怒、舌红苔黄、大便秘结，可选用天麻、菊花、夏枯草、羚羊角、决明子、干芦荟以平肝降火。肾精亏虚者如耳鸣如蝉叫、多梦健忘、腰酸膝软、遗精滑泄、舌淡苔白、大便干结，可选用枸杞子、山药、阿胶、酸枣仁、芡实、莲子肉、龟板、鹿角胶以补肾养肝，但要避免过服。气血虚弱者如面色淡白、唇白、活动后气短、劳累懒言、心慌、大便稀软、舌淡边有齿痕等，可选用党参、黄芪、龙眼肉、芡实、大枣、炒扁豆、薏米、粳米以健脾益气。气滞血瘀者如情绪郁闷之后出现头晕伴有头痛、面色晦暗、唇甲青紫、皮肤暗黄、舌暗有瘀斑、舌底部脉络迂曲等，可选用三七、桃仁、红花、老葱、白芷等以理气活血化瘀。痰浊蒙上者如头重昏蒙伴视物旋转，胸闷恶心、食少喜睡、大便溏薄不畅、舌苔白腻、晨起口苦口腻，可选择茯苓、白术、薏苡仁、陈皮、天麻、砂仁、豆蔻、郁金、生姜等健脾化湿化痰，伴口苦者可选择炒黄连、莲子心等化痰郁、清心火。

20.Tips about hypertension

Q: How can I monitor my blood pressure properly when staying at home?

A: It is crucial to monitor blood pressure regularly to help detect fluctuations and give the data to the doctor as a basis for medication adjustment. The latest international guidelines recommend using electronic sphygmomanometers to measure blood pressure, and measurements should be taken in a calm state after 30 minutes of rest and averaged over three measurements. Generally, blood pressure measured at the brachial artery is the main reference, so it is better to use an arm blood pressure monitor. Read the instructions carefully when using it, and use the cuff according to device instructions. When you first start hypertension treatment, or if you have just adjusted the dosage of medication, you should take measurements every day after waking up (before eating) and before going to bed, until your blood pressure has been stable for at least 1 week. Then, measurement frequency can be reduced. For patients with well-controlled blood pressure, take measurements once or twice a week at a time when your blood pressure is typically higher in the day, usually after waking up in the morning.

Q: How to take care of the dietary preferences of hypertensive patients when staying at home?

A: Avoid dietary indiscipline: Avoid overly fatty, sweet and salty food; daily salt intake per person should not exceed 6 grams (one beer bottle cap); pay attention to the intake of hidden salt, such as preserved vegetables, chicken essence and soy sauce. Quit smoking and drinking: Smoking can damage the vasculature, leading to qi deficiency and blood stasis, which can cause the meridians to become unstable and obstructed; alcohol can affect the transportation of spleen qi and cause phlegm to generate inside, both of which can cause fluctuations in blood pressure and the occurrence and aggravation of vertigo symptoms. In *Compendium of Materia Medica*, there is the following quote: "Eat cool foods in spring and cold foods in summer to nourish yang qi; eat warm foods in autumn and hot foods in winter to nourish yin qi." In spring and summer, yang is the most abundant. So, it is advisable to eat cool and cold foods to suppress the hyperactivity of yang and avoid hurting yin; in autumn and winter, yin is the most abundant. So, it is advisable to eat warm and hot foods to suppress the abundance of yin and protect the yang qi. After the Beginning of Autumn, the diet should begin to slowly transition to laying the foundation for the cold autumn and winter. Summer is for growing, and autumn is for harvesting. After the Beginning of Autumn, the environment gradually changes from moist to dry, so overly dry and hot, pungent products such as ginger, pepper, peppercorn, and cinnamon should be avoided in the diet, as they can easily hurt yin. Instead, consume neutral, cool and moisten foods that are sweet or sour, such as honey, lily bulb , grapes and grapefruit.

Q: How can patients with hypertension exercise and control their weight while staying at home?

A: Do physical exercises to improve your physique: Regular moderate intensity exercise such as brisk walking, Tai Chi, and Baduanjin for 30 minutes every day, 5–7 times a week, has a direct effect on lowering blood pressure and alleviating symptoms of vertigo. A decrease in systolic blood pressure of 4–9 mmHg can be achieved. Obese people should also continue to try to lose weight while staying at home: Many obese people experience dampness and phlegm, which can also be concomitant with spleen deficiency. The inability of the spleen and stomach to transport and transform leads them to brew dampness and form phlegm, which then blocks the flow of qi and blood. This can trigger the rise of clear qi, and the occurrence of dizziness and other symptoms. The systolic blood pressure reduction achieved by weight control can be up to 5–20 mmHg/10 kg weight loss. The general requirements are BMI<24 kg/m^2, waist circumference<90 cm (male) and <85 cm (female). Avoid prolonged sitting or lying down.

Q: *Why should patients with hypertension remain emotionally stable and balance work with rest?*

A: When staying at home, hypertensive patients should pay special attention to maintaining emotional stability and preventing internal injuries; happiness, anger, sadness, fear and other emotions can all hurt the internal organs. For example, anger can cause liver wind; long–term depression can deplete and damage the heart and kidney, lead to yin qi deficiency, and then cause dizziness, tinnitus and anxiety, which can manifest as blood pressure fluctuations, and even possibly a stroke caused by hypertension. Therefore, keeping a calm and positive mood can avoid fluctuations in blood pressure and control the progression of the disease. Overwork affects the nervous system's ability to regulate blood pressure, and staying up late may disrupt the sympathetic and parasympathetic nervous systems, leading to blood pressure fluctuations. According to TCM, overwork injures yin blood and qi, and the deficiency of yin blood is concomitant with the hyperactivity of yang, while qi deficiency will cause phlegm and fluid retention, which results in vertigo. Therefore, we advocate for a combination of mental and physical labor, avoiding overwork and staying up late.

Q: My blood pressure fluctuates during the change of season between summer and autumn. How can I adjust my sleep schedule when staying at home?

A: In autumn, you should start to collect the yang qi in your body, extend your sleep time compared to that in spring and summer, and collect your spirit and energy through sufficient sleep to moderate the chillness of autumn. Adequate sleep can facilitate endocrine and hormonal regulation and help stabilize blood pressure. For patients with hypertension, if you cannot sleep well even after looking for the cause and regulating your emotions, it is recommended that you take sleep aids or TCM to improve your sleep. It is recommended that you fall asleep before 22:00 daily, avoid staying up late, while ensuring that you get at least 7 hours and no more than 9 hours of sleep daily.

Q: How to properly use TCM as tea when staying at home?

A: Patients with hypertension who can visit a hospital outpatient department can be diagnosed using symptom differentiation by a TCM physician and prescribed Chinese herbal medicine to regulate the balance between yin and yang, to replenish deficiency and reduce excess, thus lowering blood pressure and alleviating symptoms. If you are unable to visit the hospital regularly or stick to taking medication, you can choose some common medications to drink as tea or grind the powder and take it with warm water daily in appropriate amounts.

The keys to selecting medication as tea substitutes are as follows. Those with liver hyperactivity of yang, manifesting as red face, pain and swelling in the head and eyes, irritability, red tongue with yellow coating, constipation, can choose tianma, chrysanthemum, selfheal, antelope horn, cassia seed, and dried aloe to calm the liver and lower the fire. Those with kidney deficiency manifesting as tinnitus like cicadas, dreamy and forgetful, lumbago and knee weakness, spermatorrhea, pale tongue with white coating, and dry stool, can choose barbary wolfberry fruit, Chinese yam, ass hide glue, spine date seed, gorgon fruit, lotus seed, tortoiseshell and deer-horn glue to nourish the liver but should avoid overdose. Those with weak qi and blood, manifesting as pale face, white lips, shortness of breath after activity, laziness and not wanting to talk after extraneous activities, panic, thin and soft stools, and pale tongue with teeth marks, can choose tangshen, milkvetch root, longan aril, gorgon fruit, Chinese-date, fried lentils, barley, japonica rice to strengthen the spleen and benefit qi. Those with qi stagnation and blood stasis, manifesting as dizziness after emotional depression with headache, dull face, bluish lips and nails, jaundice, dark tongue with petechiae, and tortuous veins at the base of the tongue, can choose sanqi, peach seed, safflower, old scallion and dahurian angelica root to regulate qi and activate blood stasis. Those with phlegm mist, manifesting with heavy head and doziness with spinning vision, chest tightness and nausea, little appetite and lethargy, loose stools, white tongue with greasy coating, bitter and greasy taste in the mouth when waking up in the morning, can choose Poria cocos, largehead atractylodes rhizome, coix seed, dried tangerine peel, tianma, fructus amoni, cardamun, turmeric root tuber and ginger to strengthen the spleen and resolve dampness and phlegm. For those also with bitterness in the mouth, choose fried goldthread rhizomes and lotus plumules to resolve phlegm and clear heart fire.

第二部分

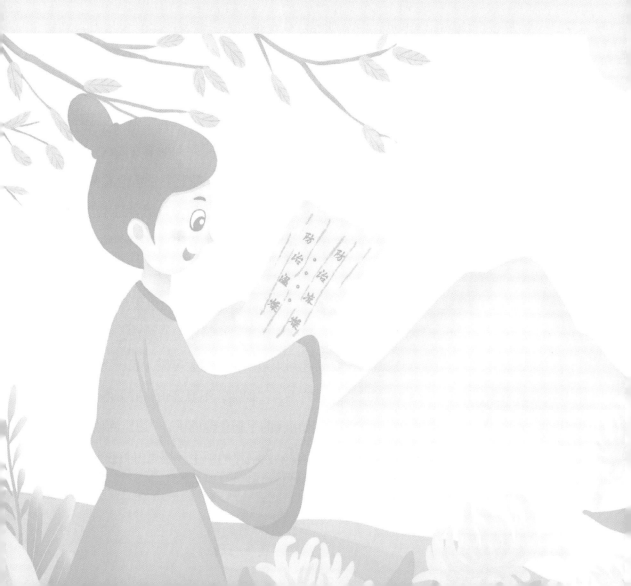

1、特殊的握手

握手，彼此伸手相互握住，是一种礼节。在电视屏幕中，领导人见面时握手象征的是一种和平合作；在日常生活中，两个人第一次见面时的握手是一种认识你很开心的表达，两个人分开离别时的握手是一种不舍的表达，两个人久别重逢时的握手是一种欣喜的表达。生活中，在不同的情景下，赋予了握手不一样的定义。

你见过这样的握手吗？一个穿着白色衣服的人，戴着严实的 N95 口罩和帽子，遮住了颜容，看不清脸上的皱褶，只能看到鱼尾纹和抬头纹，双手都戴着手套，右手环抱着对方的右手，四指紧贴着他的掌心，拇指放在他的"虎口处"，这是中医合谷穴的位置，按摩此处，有镇静止痛、疏经活络等作用，左手环抱着对方右手的掌背及手腕，拇指搭在对方桡动脉处，感受跳动的节奏。

这样特殊的握手发生在我们病房的某一刻，一个看上去瘦小但有些倔强的老头，张口用力呼吸着，看似有些急促，露着被烟熏过的参差不齐的牙齿，枕头上还留着许多脱落的头发，有白有黑，有长有短，不难看出这是一个肿瘤晚期的患者。

由于呼吸衰竭，他接受了综合治疗，刚拔除气管插管，由于痰比较多，加上身体虚弱，患者不太能主动咳痰，"医生快来，患者不配合咳痰，喉咙口有呼啦呼啦的声音。"护士喊道，我立刻赶到床边，由于职业习惯，我一下就站在患者的右侧，用一种特殊的方式握着他的手，"加油，不要害怕，好好咳嗽，你可以的，不要怕痛，我给你按摩穴位。"我用我的手握住他的手，一边监测他的脉搏，一边给他按摩穴位放松，让他在这个没有家人陪伴的陌生环境里好好恢复，随后，一口浓痰随着他努力咳嗽排出，我立刻拍了拍他的手背说道："辛苦了。"他似乎呼吸平静些了，一字一字慢慢地说道："你的手套太厚了，下次握手不要戴了，今天我很开心。"

一次特殊的握手，是一次特殊的治疗，也许比药物和器械辅助治疗对他来说更重要，虽然隔着手套，触觉上稍减弱些，但是我想只有在那时，戴着口罩、帽子、手套，才能赋予这次握手特殊的意义。等好了出院时，我们约定脱出手套再次握手，不知道以哪种形式进行，期待再次握手。

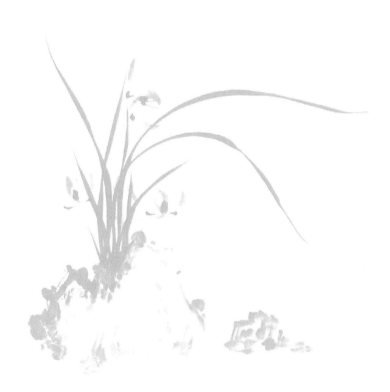

1.Special handshake

Handshake, reaching out and holding each other is a kind of etiquette. On the TV screen, the handshake symbolizes peace and cooperation when leaders meet. In daily life, when two people meet for the first time, the handshake is a happy expression of knowing you; when two people go apart,the handshake is an expression of the reuctance; when two people meet again for a long time, the handshake is an expression of joy. In life, in different situations, handshakes are given a different definition.

Have you ever seen a handshake like this? A man dressed in white, wearing a tight N95 mask and a cap that covered his face, where the only discernible part of his face were his crow's feet and forehead wrinkles. Both of his hands were wearing gloves. His right hand covered the other person's right hand, where the four fingers tightly pressed onto the other's palm with his thumb on the other's "tiger's mouth", which is the location of the acupuncture point Hegu in TCM and massaging it can relieve pain and improve circulation. His left hand wrapped around the back of the other's right palm and wrist, with his thumb lightly pressing onto the other's radial artery, feeling the rhythm of the pulse.

This special handshake occurred at the moment in our ward. An old man who looked thin but stubborn opened his mouth and breathed hard, seeming to be a little rush, showing his uneven teeth that had been smoked, and there were still many on the pillow. The hair loss was white or black, long and short. It is not difficult to see that this is a patient with an advanced tumor.

The patient underwent a comprehensive treatment for respiratory failure, and his tracheal tube was just removed. He had an accumulation of phlegm, and due to physical weakness, he was not actively coughing the phlegm up. "Come quickly doctor! The patient does not cooperate with sputum production, and there is rattling sound from his throat," the nurse shouted. I immediately rushed to the bedside. Out of professional habits, I stood on the right side of the patient right away and held his hand in a special way. "Come on! Don't be afraid. Cough up. You can do it. Don't be afraid of the pain. I will massage your point." I held his hand with mine, monitoring his pulse while massaging his acupuncture point to relax him. Holding his right hand with both of my hands despite of the thick gloves, I hoped that he could recover well in this unfamiliar environment absent of his family. A mouthful of thick phlegm was coughed out with his efforts, I patted the back of his hand and said, "Hard work." His breath seemed to be calmer. "Your gloves are too thick. Don't wear them next time when holding my hand. I am very happy today," he said slowly, word by word.

A special handshake was a special treatment that may be more important to him than medication and machine-assisted treatment. Although the sense of touch was slightly weakened through the gloves, I think only then, wearing masks, hats and gloves, to give this handshake a special meaning. When we were discharged from the hospital, we agreed to take off the gloves and shake hands again.

2、病房里的约束手套和约定

约束手套，从字面上看似乎有些冰冷，常常与"捆绑""软禁""虐待"这些词同时出现，带有一些负面色彩。然而我们医生的约束手套有着不一样的功能，常常带给我们一些特殊的感受。

这是一个暴风雨刚过的傍晚，透过窗户往外看，天空中出现了一道美丽的彩虹，病房十分安静，没有机器的报警声，也没有患者痛苦的呻吟声。在这之前，病房里有一位已过耄耋之年的奶奶，留着一头乌黑浓密的头发，她是一位有着十多年肿瘤病史的"抗癌明星"，肿瘤复发过三次，这是她第四次复发，再次接受手术治疗。奶奶本身就有消化性溃疡病史，在术后出现严重的消化道出血，身上布满了救命的管子，胃管、尿管、动脉监测导管、深静脉导管等，伴随着恶心反胃的动作，她显得十分不安及躁动，大喊大叫。她的手不由自主地活动，我一手抚摸着她的额头，说："奶奶，不要乱动，我们正在给您用药，马上就好了，放松，别紧张。我们给您戴一个有神奇作用的手套，您会慢慢好的。"同时护士已经将我们的约束手套给奶奶戴好了，用布绳宽松地固定在床边，让手不会碰及重要的"救命稻草"。这个手套像极了乒乓球拍，头部有个开口，我们可以通过此口连接血氧饱和度探头。

"没那么难受了吧，您女儿在外面等您，只要不出血了，我们就回家，戴上这个乒乓球拍，我们先熟悉一下手感，等好了，陪您用这个球拍打乒乓球。"我一边说着，一边用手调整"乒乓球拍"与奶奶手的位置，"奶奶这样握拍合适吗？"伴随着床边的安抚、及时的药物与多功能约束手套的使用，奶奶慢慢安静下来了，此时这个多功能手套与她融合在一起了，显得那么自然和谐，暴风雨也停了，从窗外看天空下的彩虹是那么美。

　　此时，一副多功能约束手套显得不那么冰冷了，带着一些温暖和谐的气息，就像经历过暴风雨后天空会挂起美丽的彩虹，同时也给我带来了一次不同寻常的约定，希望奶奶的病能快快好起来，"肿瘤君，滚蛋吧！不要阻止我和奶奶的约定，我们会用乒乓球拍拍走你。"

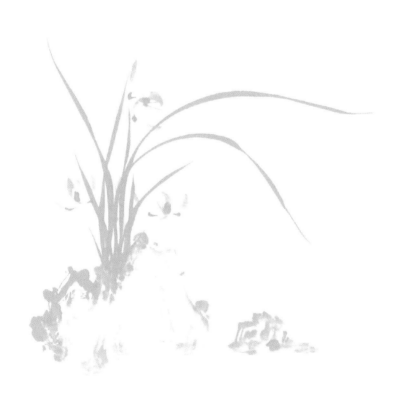

2.Restraint gloves and appointments in the ward

Literally, the restraint gloves appear to be slightly cold, and they often appear at the same time as the words "bundle" "house arrest" and "abuse", with some negative colors. However, the restraint gloves of our doctors have different functions and often give us some special feelings.

It was a stormy evening. Looking out the window, a beautiful rainbow appeared in the sky. The ward was very quiet, without the alarm of the machine, and there was no painful groan from the patient. Prior to this, there was a grandmother in the ward who was over 80 years old with black and thick hair. She was an anticancer star with a history of more than 10 years of cancer. She had tumor recurrence three times, and this was her fourth time. She had to receive surgical treatment again. The grandmother had a history of gastrointestinal ulcers, and she had severe gastrointestinal bleeding after surgery. Her body was covered with life-saving tubes, such as gastric tubes, urinary tubes, arterial monitoring catheters, and deep venous catheters. She appeared to be very restless and yelled, and her hands were moving involuntarily. I stroked her forehead with one hand and said, "Grandma, do not move. We are giving you medicine. It will be ready soon. Relax. Do not be nervous. You wear a glove that has a magical effect, and you will slowly get better." At the same time, the nurse has already put our restraint gloves on the grandma and fixed it loosely by the bed with a cloth string so that the hand will not touch the important ones. This glove is like a ping-pong racket. There is an opening on the head through which the blood oxygen saturation probe can be connected to the patient.

"It's not that uncomfortable. Your daughter is waiting for you outside. As long as there is no bleeding, we will go home and put on this table tennis racket." While speaking, I adjusted the position of the "table tennis bat" and grandma's hand by hand, "Is it suitable for you to hold the bat like this?" With the timely use of medications and multifunctional restraint gloves, the grandmother gradually calmed down. At this time, this multifunctional glove merged with her and seemed so natural and harmonious, and the storm stopped. From the window, the rainbow under the sky is beautiful.

At that moment, the pair of multifunctional restraint gloves seemed less cold, and became rather warm and harmonious, just like the beautiful rainbow that arose after the storm. It also made a pact between the grandma and me. I hope that she will get better quickly, "Go away tumor! Don't get in the way of my pact with the grandma. We will slap you away with the ping pong rackets."

3、暑气炎蒸，更惜分阴

正值大暑，大雨时行，又到了我值班之日。一切如常的行程，出地铁站时，我顿时感觉一阵暑气迎面而来。到了值班室，我换好了一身洗手服、戴好口罩帽子、用七步洗手法正确洗手后，准备好这次值班，这是我一个新的开始。

"请至9床，外科术后腹腔感染，心率快……"我放下电话，开始投入工作。到了床边，监护仪显示心脏快速跳动、血压高，指末氧饱和度90；患者略显烦躁，外科医生简要介绍病史，同时我开始与患者沟通，了解到他肚子非常疼痛，害怕进入监护室，四周环绕着的机器的运作声音和间断的报警声音令他不安。"请放心，我一直在你身边，家里人在外面等你，恢复了就会转回普通病房，不用担心。"我对他说，同时用纸巾为他擦拭眼角的泪水，他用眨眼表示同意，我握着他的手，想通过这输送一些能量。

然后，我立刻开始为他进行吸氧、留置腹腔引流管反复冲洗、有创动脉监测、输注抗感染药物等操作，当我为他进行桡动脉留置动脉导管时，我发现他的手上全是老茧，皮肤黝黑，强壮的手臂满是岁月留下的痕迹。他是我见过最配合的患者，穿刺针穿过皮肤的那一瞬间，会有一些疼痛，很多人会回避，导致穿刺失败，但他纹丝不动，我不知道是怎样的经历会让他这样。

随着指标的稳定，我到门口找家属进一步详细了解病史，"9床家属在吗？"在监护室连廊的一个角落，我看到一个年轻女孩斜挎着背包蹲在角落里低头抱着膝盖哭泣着，旁边放着日常需要的生活用品，"在这，"她带着哭声立刻站起来倚靠着墙回复，"我的父亲是个苦命人，从我出生后，一直在外做苦力。我大学毕业后在上海有了份稳定收入，有了自己的房子，今年原本打算接父亲来享福时，他被查出了肿瘤，刚开完刀，术后才两个月，前几天又出现了腹痛，可能腹腔里有感染……"我告诉她目前患者病情相对平稳，让她不要哭了，要坚强，此时只有墙和我的话能给她支持了。我强忍着在眼眶里打转的泪水，我知道我是医生，为了让她坚强、给她力量，我忍着。

安抚好家属后，我再次回到病房，"你放心，我和你女儿已经说过了，她让你好好养病，不要担心，她等你出院，现在你好好休息，其他事交给我，你放心。"我对他说道。虽然他比较虚弱，无法发出声音，但是在他的眉目之间流露出感谢之意，这对于我来说就够了。

一天忙碌而充实地过去了，我已经完成交接班。又是一天暑气炎蒸，不一样的是我多了一份感悟——珍惜与家人相处陪伴之时，珍惜每分每秒，给予为我们操劳一辈子的父母多一份关心，少留遗憾。在父母心中，无论他们身处何种境遇，甚至在生命垂危之时，放不下的永远是孩子。

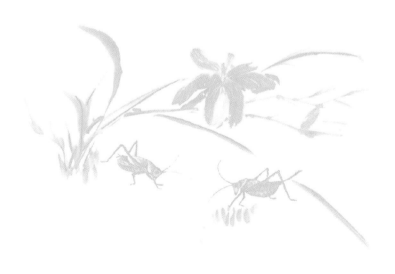

3.Summer heat steams, more cherish every monent

It was during the heat and rain, and it was the day when I was on duty again. Everything went as usual, and when I left the subway station, I suddenly felt a burst of heat oncoming. When I arrived at the duty room, I changed into a hand−washing suit, put on a mask and a hat, and washed my hands correctly, and then I was ready for the duty. This was a new start for me.

"Please go to bed 9, after surgery, abdominal infection, fast heart rate..." When I arrived at the bedside, the monitor showed rapid heartbeat, high blood pressure, and terminal oxygen saturation of 90. The patient was slightly irritable, and the surgeon briefly introduced the medical history. At the same time, I started to communicate with the patient and learned that his stomach was very painful, and he was afraid of entering the intensive care unit. He was disturbed by the sound of the operation of the machine and the intermittent alarm sound. "Please rest assured, I have been by your side. The family is waiting for you outside. When you recover, you will be transferred back to the general ward. Do not worry." I said to him and wiped the tears from the corner of his eye with a tissue, and he blinked and agreed. I shook his hand and wanted to send some energy through it.

He was immediately subjected to operations such as oxygen inhalation, indwelling peritoneal drainage tube, repeated irrigation, invasive arterial monitoring, and infusion of anti−infective drugs. His dark and strong arms are full of traces left by years on his body. He is the most cooperative patient I have ever seen. The moment the puncture needle passes through the skin, there will be some pain, which many people will avoid, resulting in puncture failure, but he does not move. I don't know what kind of experience will make him like this.

With the stability of the indicators, I went to the door to find the family members to further understand the medical history. "Are the family members of the bed 9?" She was crying on her knees, with daily necessities placed next to her. "Here," she immediately stood up and leaned against the wall with a cry of crying, "my father is a hard worker. Since I was born, he have been working outside. After graduating from college, I had a stable income in Shanghai and had my own house. When I was planning to take my father to enjoy good fortune, he was diagnosed with a tumor. Just after the surgery, he had abdominal pain a few days after the surgery. Maybe there is an infection in the abdominal cavity..." I told her that her father's condition was relatively stable, so she should not cry and be strong. At this time, only the wall and my words can support her. Knowing that I am a doctor, I endure to make her strong and give her strength.

After comforting the family members, I went back to the ward again, saying, "Don't worry. I have already told your daughter, and she told you to take care of your illness, and don't worry. She is waiting for you to be discharged. Now you have a good rest, and leave the rest to me. Don't worry," I said to him. Although he is relatively weak and unable to make a sound, the expression of gratitude between his eyebrows is enough for me.

After a busy and fulfilling day, I completed the handover. It was another day of heat and heat, and the difference was that I had an extra feeling—to cherish the time when I was with my family, to cherish every minute and every second, and to give more care and less regret to the parents who have worked for us for a lifetime. In the minds of parents, no matter what kind of situation they are in or even when their lives are dying, it is always the children who cannot let go.

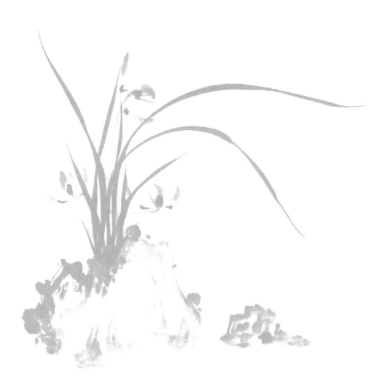

4. 听诊器的故事

经过一天烈日的蒸烤，地表温度已经高达40 ℃，大家的心理已经烦躁不安，病房似乎经历了一次"大洗牌"，床上躺着不同的面孔，交班有序进行着。"医生，新患者由急诊科转入……"护士一边接听着电话，一边喊道。此刻时间停顿30秒，突然大家都不说话了，最尴尬的事情出现了，在交班过程中来了患者。

伴随着转运车的声音，患者来了，大家立刻围上去，按照平时的标准动作过床、吸氧、连接心电监护。我到了病床边，那是一位白发苍苍、胸前皮下还隐约着有一枚"勋章"的爷爷，一看心电监护，本能的反应是那枚东西是心脏永久起搏器。为了判断意识及症状，我喊道："生命体征平稳，爷爷，您知道在哪吗？"老爷爷没有回答，但是眼睛在不停地转动，似乎要表达什么，嘴巴里发出模糊不清的声音，带着一点北方的乡音，但是我听不太清楚，我明白了，他可能得了老年人常有的"耳聋"，我特意俯身下去对着他的耳朵大声说："您知道在哪里吗？您是不是听不清？"他点头回应道："是的。"

此时，在我身边的一位经验丰富的"老医生"出场了，她拿着听诊器听筒，我第一反应是她要听诊，我连忙说我来。结果她把听头给爷爷戴上，她对着听筒大声说道："这样好一点吗？"爷爷开心地说："非常清楚。"他脸上露出了笑容，并仔细地描述了他的症状，经过一系列针对性处理后，爷爷慢慢睡着了。事后我们与家属联系上，知道爷爷听力不好，这几天在其他医院也没怎么睡，一直不舒服。

一个听诊器除了可以帮助医生完成重要的听诊检查外，在某些情况下，还可以成为与患者沟通的桥梁。如果一直处于听不清周围声音的情况下，患者会感觉到恐惧烦躁，可能会导致病情恶化，一次仔细的观察可能会使问题迎刃而解。临床医生正如其名字一样，需要站在床边仔细观察患者，包括对看似普通的患者进行听力、视力评估。

听诊器发明已有近 200 年的历史，从法国医生雷奈克为了诊治患者，第一次提出听诊器的概念，到吴孟超院士在冬天查房用双手先捂热听诊器再为患者听诊，到为了能让患者听清楚，发现听诊器的新用途，在听诊器的故事中，不同的主人公、不同的场景，但伴随着的都是那一份来自医生的爱，一份给予患者希望的爱。此时我的脑海中浮现了美国医生特鲁多曾经对医生这个职业的一段非常著名的描述："有时是治愈，常常是帮助，总是去安慰。"

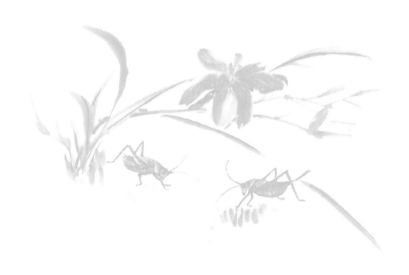

4.The story of the stethoscope

It was an extremely hot day, with the sun grilling and surface temperature over 40 ℃. We were rather restless. The ward had undergone a "reshuffle", with different faces on the beds, but the change of shift was still in order. "Doctor, a new patient will be transferred from the emergency department here..." The nurse shouted as she answered the call. Time instantly froze, and for 30 seconds everyone was silent. The most awkward thing happened — in the process of a shift handover there came a new patient.

Accompanied by the sound of the transfer vehicle, the patient came, and everyone immediately surrounded the bed, inhaled oxygen, and connected to the ECG monitoring according to the usual standard actions. The grandfather, who had a vague "medal". I looked at the ECG monitoring and instinctively reflected that the thing was a permanent pacemaker. To determine the consciousness and symptoms, I yelled, "Vital signs are stable. Grandpa, do you know where?" The grandfather did not answer, but his eyes kept turning as if to express something, and his mouth made a vague voice. He had a little northern accent, but I could not hear clearly. I understood that he might have the "deafness" that the elderly often have. I leaned over and said loudly to his ear, "Do you know where it is? Are you inaudible?" He nodded and replied, "Yes."

At this time, an experienced "old doctor" next to me showed up, holding the stethoscope earpiece. My first reaction was that she wanted to auscultate, and I quickly said, "I'm here." As a result, she brought the earpiece to the grandpa, and she said loudly into the earpiece: "Is this better?" Grandpa said happily: "Very clear." There was a smile on his face and a detailed description of his symptoms. After a series of targeted treatments, the grandpa fell asleep slowly. Afterward, we contacted the family members and learned that the grandpa had poor hearing and did not sleep much in other hospitals these days.

In addition to helping doctors complete important auscultation examinations, a stethoscope can also become a bridge for communication with patients in some cases. If the patient is always in a situation where he or she cannot hear the surrounding sounds, the patient will feel fear and irritability, which may lead to the deterioration of the condition. Careful observation may easily solve the problem. As the name suggests, the clinician needs to stand by the bedside to observe the patient carefully, including hearing and visual acuity assessment for seemingly ordinary patients.

The stethoscope has been invented for nearly 200 years. From the French doctor Rene Laennec, who first proposed the concept of the stethoscope to treat patients to academician Mengchao Wu, who warmed up the stethoscope with his hands before listening to patients in winter, to this senior doctor who used the stethoscope today to let the patient hear clearly and showed me a new way to use the stethoscope, in each story of the stethoscope, the tasks and scenarios are different, but the stethoscope always conveys the love from doctors. A love that gives hope to the patients. I am reminded of a very famous quote from the American doctor Edward Livingston Trudeau describing our profession: "To cure sometimes, to relieve often, and to comfort always."